Supervision for Occupational Therapy

Supervision for Occupational Therapy is a practical text that guides both supervisors and supervisees to make the most out of supervision opportunities.

While supervision in occupational therapy is vital as a mechanism for public and professional safety, learning how to do it successfully on-the-job can be a daunting prospect. By gathering stories from different professions, sectors, and parts of the world, this book is a hands-on guide to help occupational therapists navigate the complexities of supervision throughout their careers. This book presents, for the first time, the 3Cs for Effective Supervision (Connections, Content, and Continuing development), which offers a platform for supervisors and supervisees to frame their supervision practices. The chapters discuss common models and theories for supervision, ideas for how to structure relationships and sessions, templates and question guides for enhancing conversations, and practical strategies for dealing with common challenges. The book also considers the impact of workforce issues, diverse populations, and regional/rural/remote practice on supervision.

Offering career-span advice and a process of self- and professional development to work through, this book provides a way to scaffold and support supervisors' and supervisees' learning and practice of supervision throughout working life. It is an essential guide for all occupational therapists.

The eResources for this book are available at www.Routledge.com/9780367552428.

Karina Dancza (she/her/hers) is an occupational therapy educator who has worked in practice with children and young people, in policy and academic roles. Karina is passionate about translating knowledge for practical application and the education of current and future professionals. She has worked extensively in her various roles to support workforce development through education, continuing professional development, and, of course, supervision. Australian-born, her postgraduate working life so far has consisted of stints in Australia, England, Wales, and Singapore. These changes are intentional, as connecting with different people and viewpoints is what makes life so interesting.

Anita Volkert (she/her/hers) is an occupational therapy educator. Having worked in clinical practice, management, professional facilitation, and development, policy, and education roles, Anita is interested in workforce development and support. She has spent many years supervising and mentoring others, and being supervised, mentored, and occasionally coached. Anita is particularly interested in exploring ways to ensure that future occupational therapists and health professionals can sustain long, exciting, and rewarding careers in the dynamic and changing health and social care environment – and supervision is one of those ways.

Stephanie Tempest (she/her/hers) is an occupational therapist. Her other work roles include health professional, supervisor, coachee, strategic leader, author, critical friend, and business owner. Of equal, if not greater, importance are the meaningful occupations associated with roles including, but not limited to, being a mum, partner, friend, daughter, sister, colleague, and puppy-owner. Stephanie continues to seek opportunities to actively learn about the impact that her dominant and marginalised identities have on her ability to engage in supervision and personal/professional development, appreciating that we are all work in progress.

Supervision for Occupational Therapy

Practical Guidance for Supervisors and Supervisees

Edited by
Karina Dancza, Anita Volkert, and
Stephanie Tempest

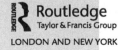

Routledge
Taylor & Francis Group

LONDON AND NEW YORK

First published 2023
by Routledge
4 Park Square, Milton Park, Abingdon, Oxon OX14 4RN

and by Routledge
605 Third Avenue, New York, NY 10158

Routledge is an imprint of the Taylor & Francis Group, an informa business

British Library Cataloguing-in-Publication Data
A catalogue record for this book is available from the British Library

ISBN: 978-0-367-55242-8 (hbk)
ISBN: 978-0-367-55236-7 (pbk)
ISBN: 978-1-003-09254-4 (ebk)

DOI: 10.4324/9781003092544

Typeset in Garamond
by SPi Technologies India Pvt Ltd (Straive)

To all the supervisors and supervisees who are striving to make a difference.

Contents

Figures

Tables

Boxes

⬇ Appendices

Chapter authors

Joanne M. Baird (she/her/hers) is an occupational therapist and associate professor at the University of Pittsburgh, USA. Joanne has been an educator for her entire career, working to develop student programmes and mentor junior practitioners in the clinic before working as an associate professor. Her interest in supervision is fuelled by its intrinsic link to teaching and learning and the importance of ever-evolving and dynamic approaches to communication and problem-solving.

Jodie Copley (she/her/hers) is an associate professor of occupational therapy at the University of Queensland, Australia. Jodie's main drive as a clinician and educator for more than 30 years has been to contribute to high-quality occupational therapy for clients by providing supervision to hundreds of occupational therapy students and practitioners. Jodie believes that the process of supervision is as much about the learning of the supervisor as the supervisee, so doing supervision well is a 'win–win' for everyone.

Vicki Craig (she/her/hers) is a qualified counsellor and an accredited member of the British Association for Counselling and Psychotherapy. Engaging with supervision is an integral part of her work. She values the environment of high support and challenge that can be created within a supervisory relationship. She wholeheartedly believes that effective supervision benefits both her professional and personal relationships as it affords a protective space for self-reflection.

Christine Craik (she/her/hers) is an occupational therapist based in London. Throughout her long career as a practitioner, manager, educator, and researcher, Christine has endeavoured to enable other occupational therapists to develop their potential. Supervision is a key element of this. It provides the supervisor with a valuable learning opportunity and the reward of seeing others progress in their careers. More importantly, it improves and extends the intervention delivered to the people we serve.

Cate Fitzgerald (she/her/hers) is an occupational therapist currently in a leadership role supporting the quality of student and new graduate education within health workplaces. She enjoys contributing to the clinical education of health professionals for the people they work with and for. Seeking evidence and perspectives on how supervision supports professional practice is a passion as she has seen the difference quality supervision can make to the practice and wellbeing of occupational therapists.

Sarah Harvey (she/her/hers) is an occupational therapist and course director at Canterbury Christ Church University, UK. Sarah is interested in the creativity that occurs when individuals are given time to reflect and discuss their everyday practice in both dyadic and group contexts. She believes that supervision provides a wonderful space for reflexivity, analysis, and strategic development within occupational therapy practice.

Priya Martin (she/her/hers) is an occupational therapist and a senior research fellow at the University of Queensland, Australia. Priya is a health services researcher and a health professions educator with an interest in improving the safety and quality of healthcare. She is an internationally recognised leader in the practice and research of clinical supervision. She has contributed to supervision literature through her award-winning PhD and postdoctoral studies. Her professional commitment and excellence have been recognised through 17 prestigious awards and prizes to date.

Áine O'Dea (she/her/hers) is a consultant occupational therapist at Radiance Consulting, Ireland. Áine provides management consultancy and external clinical supervision for occupational therapists. Áine is passionate about enhancing managers' and occupational therapists' capacity to reason from a professional, evidence-informed, and policy perspective. In addition, she helps occupational therapists to translate their professional knowledge and research evidence into practice.

Merrolee Penman (she/her/hers) is an occupational therapist and associate professor at Curtin University and research affiliate at The University of Sydney, Australia, whose research and practice interests centre on learning – whether that be of therapists in practice or students during their degrees. Merrolee's interest in supervision stems from her observations of the therapist–student dyad during practice education placements. Her research has centred on co-developing, with educators, models of supervisory practice that support students' capacity to be effective self-regulating learners.

Chapter contributors

Wendy H. Ducat (she/her/hers) is a clinical psychologist and program manager at Queensland Centre for Mental Health Learning, West Moreton Health, Australia.

Jenniffer García Rojas (she/her/hers) is an occupational therapist and PhD candidate at the University of Queensland, Australia and academic at Universidad del Desarrollo in Chile.

Charmaine Green (she/her/hers) is a PhD scholar and a senior researcher at WA Centre for Rural Health, UWA, Australia.

Helen Hak (she/her/hers) is a strategic clinical lead occupational therapist for stroke, United Kingdom.

Naureen Javed Hirani (she/her/hers) is a director of research and development at the AMI School, Junior Section, Pakistan.

Carol-Ann Howson (she/her/hers) is a senior lecturer in social work at the University of Hertfordshire, United Kingdom.

Susan E. Gilbert Hunt (she/her/hers) is an occupational therapist based in South Australia.

Samreen Jawaid (she/her/hers) is a director of research and development at the AMI School, Nursery Section, Pakistan.

Ann Kennedy-Behr (she/her/hers) is an occupational therapist in private practice and Adjunct Senior Lecturer at the University of South Australia.

Debbie Kramer-Roy (she/her/hers) is an educational director of the European MSc in Occupational Therapy at Amsterdam University of Applied Sciences, the Netherlands.

Kyrin Liong (she/her/hers) is an assistant professor of mechanical engineering with the Singapore Institute of Technology.

Suhailah Mohamed (she/her/hers) is an occupational therapist and Head of Allied Health Professions, The Chief Allied Health Professions Office for England, National Medical Directorate, NHS England.

Monica Moran (she/her/hers) is an occupational therapist and associate professor of rural health at the WA Centre for Rural Health, UWA, Australia.

Lennelle (Lenny) Patricia Papertalk (she/her/hers) is a social worker and community engagement officer at the WA Centre for Rural Health, UWA, Australia.

Madiha Sajid, FHEA (she/her/hers) is the chair of the National Network of Parents & Carers in Higher Education UK, Imperial College London, United Kingdom.

Maha Sohail (she/her/hers) is an occupational therapist with the Sindh Institute of Physical Medicine and Rehabilitation, Karachi, Pakistan.

Margaret Spencer (she/her/hers) is a consultant occupational therapy practitioner at OT360, UK.

Gillian M. Taylor (she/her/hers) is an independent occupational therapist based in south-west England.

Shamala Thilarajah (she/her/hers) is a senior principal physiotherapist with Singapore General Hospital.

Su Ren Wong (she/her/hers) is a principal occupational therapist at the National University Hospital. She is also an assistant professor at the Singapore Institute of Technology.

Esther Yuen Ling Tai (she/her/hers) is a principal occupational therapist and clinical education lead (allied health) at the National University Hospital, Singapore.

Foreword

We are delighted to introduce this new book which so clearly and comprehensively describes supervision in practice and educational settings. The authors have skillfully gathered and synthesized relevant research from management, education, organizational psychology, and occupational therapy. They present this theoretically sound material in an accessible, down-to-earth manner illustrated by artful graphics.

Writing this foreword has caused us to reflect on our own supervisory experiences. Both of us have extensive management, education, and practice on our resumes. Each has taught graduate courses on supervision in our own disciplines. Barbara has been an occupational therapy supervisor, manager, and health care administrator, followed by her academic career as a program director, faculty supervisor, teacher, and student advisor. John was a supervisor of local education programs and at state government levels. He was a supervisor of faculty and student advisor/supervisor in his academic life. From our professional and academic experiences, we really appreciate supervision that engenders safe spaces, atmospheres of trust, and emphasis on professional growth. These are on-going themes richly represented in the tapestry of this book.

We were struck by how beautifully authors attended to complexity in both the personal and cultural contexts of supervision. Cultural humility is highlighted, and then blended into effective supervision strategies. The care the authors and contributors take to be culturally authentic gives a sense of humility, sensitivity, and honesty.

Inclusion is another important thread. You, the reader, are warmly "invited" to "share" in reflective stories that richly illustrate key points of supervision. Within these stories we learn of genuine struggles and triumphs among practicing supervisors. We find this authentic and honest – engendering a sense of trust in this work.

The mindset of growth through effective supervision is another element we related to strongly. From our perspective, good supervision is a form of highly customized education. The authors provide many supervisory approaches that develop higher-level skills and the striving for excellence that benefits all service recipients. They also provide a range of practical approaches to prompt reflection.

All of the many aspects of supervision come together as the authors artfully synthesize supervision research. Then they use traditional and progressive perspectives to build their supervision framework: the 3Cs for Effective Supervision, consisting of Connections, Content and

Continuing development. We find the 3Cs approach yields a mindful, empathic, and developmental approach to effective supervision.

After presenting their emerging framework the authors and contributors move on to the practical realities of supervision. They deal with such issues as how knowledge common to occupational therapists can be applied to supervision, while carefully distinguishing the supervisory role from that of a therapy role. Additionally, they suggest approaches to the inevitable tensions that arise in supervisory roles and relationships. They expand the discussion to speak to the importance of supervision from managerial and strategic perspectives. Finally, they share their perspectives on future directions of, and needed scholarship about, supervision.

We found this book to be created on a foundation of deep research used to construct new and exciting ideas with regard to effective supervision, while also sharing reliable tried and true methods. In many ways, this text could be considered a one-stop shop for those interested in learning the complex tapestry of supervision.

One last comment: These authors are fine scholars who present their authentic selves as ones who appreciate the deep mysteries of scholarly inquiry.

> We find the more we know the more we realise we don't know … we find that we apply ideas more lightly and in a considered way, rather than attempting to be an expert.

This quotation exemplifies a humility that is a strong and comforting foundation of this exciting book.

John and Barbara Schell, December 2021

John W. Schell, Ph.D.,
Professor Emeritus, College of Education,
University of Georgia; co-owner, Schell Consulting

Barbara A. Boyt Schell, Ph.D., OT/L, FAOTA,
Professor Emerita, School of Occupational Therapy,
Brenau University;
co-owner, Schell Consulting

Preface

This book is the evolution of our perspectives on supervision after many years of engaging with the literature, experience as supervisors and supervisees across different sectors, and from conversations, debates, and reflections with people we admire, trust, and respect. Additionally, it has been informed by those we disagree with, and we are grateful to them for prompting us to think differently. We are passionate to see our profession reach its potential to make the impact on people's lives in a way that we know it can. But to do this requires attention, intention, and effort.

Supervision, in all its many forms, offers one of the best ways for occupational therapists to work to the top of their capabilities. It is also a mechanism that enhances professional and public safety – so important in an increasingly risk-driven world. And while supervision features in occupational therapy, we believe that we can make more of this valuable resource, embedding it as core within our profession. We offer this book as our contribution to valuing and enhancing supervision and look forward to working together to continue these conversations and turn them into practical actions and meaningful changes.

THE NEED FOR A BOOK ON SUPERVISION IN OCCUPATIONAL THERAPY

When we embarked on writing this book, the first thing that came to mind was to articulate why we felt this book was needed. We are not the first and we won't be the last people to write about supervision. Indeed, occupational therapists and other professionals have been highlighting the need for more effective supervision since at least 2001 (Sweeney et al., 2001). Yet, despite this, Fone (2006) found a lack of practical information and structured guidelines to support supervision, despite its role as an "essential component" of service delivery (p. 277). Given the time that has passed, we wondered what blockages remained to prevent the delivery of effective supervision when so many have already argued for it.

In our research for this book, the learning from our collective experiences, and discussions with many people, we are still finding there is a need for adequate and consistent support and strategies for occupational therapists to experience effective supervision. This ranges from protected time for supervision to guidance on what to do to make the most of supervisory opportunities.

Professional development to enhance our own knowledge and skills as supervisors and supervisees is also critically needed.

We are in a profession and a broader context that focuses almost exclusively on working effectively and efficiently with people who access our services. We are part of an expensive resource (a justifiable expense in our opinion). However, the link between supervision, effectiveness, and efficiency has not yet been adequately made, and this means supervision is often not prioritised in strategic service planning and delivery. Supervision thus becomes a Cinderella offering; it gets the crumbs of time and attention fitted in around other 'more important' tasks.

As we move forward in the (ever lengthening) wake and impact of the global COVID-19 pandemic, we want to raise awareness – among individual practitioners and those who make decisions about resourcing and practice – about the vital contribution that supervision can offer to protect the wellbeing of the workforce, retain talent, and ensure the delivery of high-quality and safe services for the people who need them.

HOW THE BOOK IS SET OUT

Our book is organised over ten chapters. We begin with foundational ideas (chapters 1 and 2), and then, drawing on some of this foundational work, we share how we view supervision, introducing the 3Cs for Effective Supervision (Chapter 3). Reflecting on three vital components of supervision, we explore making Connections (Chapter 4), organising Content (Chapter 5), and Continuing development of professional and supervisory knowledge and skills (Chapter 6). We then relate how we can use our occupational therapy knowledge and skills to enhance supervision (Chapter 7) and how to work through tensions when they arise in supervision (Chapter 8). Finally, we look at supervision from managerial and strategic leadership perspectives (Chapter 9) and conclude by considering how we can create change and suggest potential future directions for research and supervisory practices (Chapter 10).

Our book is evidence informed (where we have found evidence), and we have offered practical ideas to illustrate concepts. We also make suggestions where we have briefly introduced topics but recommend wider reading, as we cannot cover everything in one book. We anticipate that the ideas we present will be used as inspiration, as they will need to be adapted to the culture of your workplace and to local and national policy contexts. To assist in this process, we have included some special features throughout the book:

- **Chapter intentions** open each chapter so you can scan the main points covered and find what you're looking for.
- **Chapter highlights** offer details of the sections within the chapter.
- **Chapter resources** list the figures, boxes, and appendices associated with the chapter (where you will find many of our practical ideas for supervision).
- **Critical commentary** is presented at the end of each chapter as an alternative perspective, reflection, or critique of concepts that we found particularly interesting or troublesome.

In addition, we have been conscious to include a range of voices to contribute to the book, as our international experience tells us time and again that one size does not fit all. We are grateful to the many authors and contributors who gave their time and reflective stories as examples of their personal learning within supervision. We invite you to begin with Chapter 1 as we offer a bit more context, outlining how we use different terms and how we aim to promote inclusivity in our book and in supervision. We look forward to sharing future conversations with you (#3CSupervision).

Karina Dancza, Anita Volkert, and Stephanie Tempest

REFERENCES

Fone, S. (2006) 'Effective supervision for occupational therapists: the development and implementation of an information package', *Australian Occupational Therapy Journal*, 53(4), pp. 277–283.

Sweeney, G., Webley, P., and Treacher, A. (2001) 'Supervision in occupational therapy, part 1: the supervisor's anxieties', *British Journal of Occupational Therapy*, 64(7), pp. 337–345.

Acknowledgements

First, we would like to thank all the authors, contributors, and people who, both formally and informally, have been involved in the development of this book. Our many conversations have shaped the content and, without you, this book would not have evolved in a way which makes us both proud and grateful.

Our ideas have developed from the occupational therapists who have pioneered and championed the value of supervision over many years, and we thank you for providing a foundation on which we can build. We are also appreciative of the work undertaken in supervision from beyond our profession. We have been inspired and have drawn heavily from these ideas and perspectives.

We are grateful for the support of our publishers who have helped us along the way. Our families and friends have also made this possible, and we thank you for your patience as we stole extra moments to revise the chapters 'just one more time'.

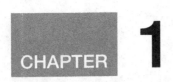

CHAPTER 1

Setting the stage for supervision

Priya Martin, Karina Dancza, Anita Volkert, and Stephanie Tempest

With contributions from Gillian M. Taylor, Wendy H. Ducat, and Jenniffer García Rojas

CHAPTER INTENTIONS

In this chapter, we invite you to:

- Review the intentions of the editors, authors, and contributors to promote inclusivity in the book and in supervision
- Explore the similarities and differences between supervision, managerial supervision, mentoring, and coaching
- Examine the purpose and function of supervision
- Reflect on the importance of creating a safe space and time for supervision
- Appraise how supervision models and frameworks can be used in practice.

CHAPTER HIGHLIGHTS

- An overview of supervision
- Addressing inclusivity in this book
- Definitions used in this book for supervision, managerial supervision, mentoring, and coaching
- Functions of supervision
- Creating a safe space and time for supervision
- Supervision frameworks and models
- Inclusive supervision
- Critical commentary: Supervision is complicated. Or is it joyful, rewarding, inspiring, and affirming … or all of the above?

DOI: 10.4324/9781003092544-1

CHAPTER RESOURCES

Figures

- Figure 1.1 The Queer People of Colour (QPOC) Resilience-Based Model of Supervision
- Figure 1.2 Cyclical Model of White Awareness

Boxes

- Box 1.1 Editor's Reflective Story: Experience of supervision
- Box 1.2 Editor's Reflective Story: Experience of managerial supervision
- Box 1.3 Editor's Reflective Story: Experience of mentoring
- Box 1.4 Editor's Reflective Story: Experience of coaching
- Box 1.5 Reflective Story by Gill Taylor: The importance of a safe space for supervision
- Box 1.6 Reflective Story by Jenniffer García Rojas: The importance of time for mentoring and supervision
- Box 1.7 Reflecting on the importance of time and a safe space for supervision
- Box 1.8 The Health and Care Professions Council (HCPC)'s rapid review of supervision questions
- Box 1.9 Critical questions when selecting a supervision framework
- Box 1.10 Connecting Practice: 13 domains of supervision
- Box 1.11 Self-reflection questions from the Queer People of Colour (QPOC) Resilience-Based Model of Supervision
- Box 1.12 Reflective questions for identity-conscious supervision
- Box 1.13 Practical tips for using a framework and/or model to frame supervision
- Box 1.14 A starting point for supporting people to share their individual needs

AN OVERVIEW OF SUPERVISION

Supervision and its underpinning concepts are not new. As an occupational therapist, it is likely that you have experienced supervision from the time you were a student. When supervision is working well, it can provide you with a sense of belonging to the profession, as well as energy, motivation to do something new, and a comfort when the work gets tough. You may, however, pay more attention to the process of supervision when you become a supervisor yourself, or if there is tension between the people involved. Whatever the reason you have decided to pick up this book, we hope that you find some useful take-aways from it.

There is a long history of doing supervision, writing about supervision, and supervision research, especially within the social work, psychology, and counselling professions where models of supervision were published in the 1970s and early 1980s (for an early example, see Kadushin, 1968). Occupational therapy has drawn on this understanding from outside our profession to develop specific guides and statements for supervision, for example the American Occupational Therapy Association (1981) and the United Kingdom's College of Occupational Therapists (1990).

Profession-specific research began to gather some momentum in the two decades that followed (for example Sweeney et al., 2001a, 2001b, 2001c). Multi-professional guidance for supervision also continues to be published (Davys et al., 2021), as new roles and ways of working develop within the healthcare system, such as for advanced practitioners (Health Education England, 2020).

This chapter provides an overview of the foundations for supervision. It is essentially a place to start if you want to know more about what supervision looks like, or if you want to begin to formulate a strategy for supervision in your own workplace. Like many processes, there is no one 'correct' way to do supervision. Being flexible to match the demands of the supervisees, supervisors, and wider context will help the process remain meaningful and beneficial. However, we do require a foundation for thinking about supervision so we can make informed decisions about what is needed, and not only rely on our own experiences of supervision or historical workplace practices.

Before we start to explore the purpose and function, the frameworks and models, and the key concepts that support supervision, it is important to clarify definitions of key terms that will feature in this book. We also wish to explain our process for addressing inclusivity in this book, and we thought this would be a good place to begin.

ADDRESSING INCLUSIVITY IN THIS BOOK

We would like to introduce ourselves as the editorial and author team and invite you to read our biographies to get a sense of who we are and the perspectives we bring to this book. We acknowledge that our dominant identities offer us privilege and safety in our profession. We are continuing to learn about the impact of both our dominant and marginalised identities and how these influence our work and the writing of this book. **If we have unintentionally used language or concepts that undermine our efforts, we would like you to let us know**. We know it is important for voices to be heard and for people to see themselves within our work and we have endeavoured to collaborate and make space for this to happen. Your feedback will help us as we continue to learn.

This book has been written at a point in time where conversations and actions around inclusivity have gained prominence in parts of the world. We have kept the content of this book under continuous review and have sought additional contributions where we identified the need to amplify voices and representation. But we recognise that **views change constantly**, and we may not always get this right.

We have consciously attempted to use respectful and inclusive language in our writing. We have discussed this with each other within the editorial team, with authors, with our publisher, and by seeking advice from available resources. For example, we have adopted **gender-neutral language** throughout this book (e.g. they/them), unless our contributors have chosen to identify themselves in a specific way.

When describing **relationships between people**, we use the terms supervisor, mentor, and coach to mean the more experienced person in the relevant field, and supervisee, mentee, and coachee to mean the person receiving guidance or support.

We have chosen to adopt the term '**people who access services**', and this includes individuals, families, carers, and groups or communities you work with in a professional capacity. This term has been adopted by the Royal College of Occupational Therapists (RCOT, 2021) in their Professional Standards for Occupational Therapy Practice, Conduct, and Ethics, as it was a term identified as acceptable from a cohort of people we serve. Other similar terms which may be found in the literature and in practice are patient, client, service user, and customer.

When we use the terms 'professionals' or 'practitioners' we refer to occupational therapists who work in any sector, including independent practice. This includes (but is not limited to) healthcare, social care, education, research, policy, leadership, and any emerging settings, e.g. prisons. As we start our journey through supervision in this book, the next area we will focus on is some of the definitions.

DEFINITIONS USED IN THIS BOOK

There are many terms and definitions used to describe supervision. In this book we are not attempting to redefine any of them. However, we do need to make clear how we intend to use these different terms. As you read, you may feel like there is overlap between them, and that is probably true. But there are some important differences too. We need to start somewhere, so we begin by outlining some commonly used terms.

Supervision

We will use 'supervision' as a broad term that describes a formal process of learning and professional development intended to promote optimal outcomes, safety, and the wellbeing of people who access services. The purpose of supervision is to:

- enhance the supervisee's knowledge, skills, and capability
- provide emotional support, and
- ensure professional and organisational standards are maintained.

Terms that also appear in the literature that could be similar include 'professional supervision' (College of Occupational Therapists, 2015; Fitzpatrick et al., 2012), or 'clinical supervision' (Occupational Therapy Australia, 2019; Martin et al., 2014). Our first Editor's **Reflective Story (Box 1.1)** shares experiences of supervision as an example.

BOX 1.1

Editor's Reflective Story: Experience of supervision

In a previous role as the professional development manager at a national professional body, I (Steph) had monthly supervision with the head of the team. Supervision was essential to help me develop my knowledge, skills, and capabilities to work at a national, strategic level. Supervision became a place where I could explore and better understand my own values and learn more about how these influenced my decisions and emotional responses. In this sense, it became a form of emotional support while ensuring my work remained aligned to the objectives set within the business plan.

'**Managerial supervision**' may share some common features with more clinically or professionally focused supervision, but there are some important differences. Managerial supervision tends to be associated with performance reviews, contributions to organisational outcomes, and compliance with workplace expectations (Snowdon, 2018). For example, managerial supervision may include:

- enhancing team relationships and dynamics
- managing performance and productivity
- human resource management (e.g. annual leave, sick leave, mandatory training), and
- caseload/workload allocation and monitoring.

Terms that also appear in the literature that could be similar include '**operational management**' (Victorian Government, 2019) or '**line management**' (Martin et al., 2014). A further challenge is that often the manager is also the supervisor, and this can create some confusion and tension. We will come back to this later, but to illustrate managerial supervision, we invite you to read our second Editor's **Reflective Story (Box 1.2)**.

BOX 1.2

Editor's Reflective Story: Experience of managerial supervision

After close to ten years working as a practitioner in children's services, I (Karina) decided to transition to a 'new' career in academia. The professional lead in the university provided managerial supervision and was responsible for reviewing teaching allocation, undertaking annual appraisal, and ensuring compliance with all mandatory training. During these managerial supervision sessions, we were able to create space to discuss my future career plans, including a desire to further my academic qualifications. Rather than leave my post to study full-time, my supervisor created the opportunity for me to study part-time for my PhD degree, while continuing to work as a lecturer. This was a mutually beneficial outcome from our managerial supervision sessions; I remained working within the service for eight years and successfully completed my postgraduate degree. In addition, for the last three years in the role, I was also able to reduce to part-time hours to take on another part-time policy role. I am very grateful for the flexibility and vision of my managerial supervisor in supporting my career choices and helping me to be the professional I am today.

To summarise, regardless of the terminology or type, **the ultimate purpose of supervision** – whether stated or implied – is to enhance the quality, safety, and effectiveness of services for the benefit of people who access them (Snowdon et al., 2016, 2017).

Mentoring

'**Mentoring**' is generally seen as "a relationship between two people where the individual with more experience, knowledge, and connections is able to pass along what they have learned to a more junior individual within a certain field. The more senior individual is the mentor, and the more junior individual is the mentee" (Oshinkale, 2019, para. 2).

Mentoring tends to focus on the development of the whole person and their future career trajectory, rather than on specific practice caseloads/workloads. Another form of mentoring which is still in relative infancy is '**reverse mentoring**', where a more junior person shares expertise with a more senior person. It has been identified as an efficient process to share knowledge, create organisational engagement, develop leadership capacity, and build intergenerational relations based on mutual respect (Gadomska-Lila, 2020).

A mentoring relationship may overlap with a supervisory relationship, or it could be two separate forms of support. It is possible, for example, for a graduate with between one and two years' experience to mentor a brand-new graduate. Both parties could also receive additional supervision.

Alternatively, a supervisor may also adopt a mentoring role in certain situations. A mentor may be external to the organisation and removed from the day-to-day activities of the mentee so that they can focus on overall career-review and planning. Often mentors have some experience in your own profession (e.g. occupational therapy) or the field you work in (e.g. research) and can offer guidance from an 'insider' perspective. Our third Editor's **Reflective Story (Box 1.3)** shares an experience of mentoring.

BOX 1.3

Editor's Reflective Story: Experience of mentoring

When I (Anita) moved into academia, I was excited but also nervous. I had worked for my entire career within statutory health services in Australia and the United Kingdom. Although I had worked my way to a relatively high level, the jump into teaching, learning, and research felt quite overwhelming. I was accustomed to supervision, but not to mentoring approaches. The institution had an arrangement whereby new staff were mentored by an experienced academic, usually from within their department (but not always, as there are some benefits to cross-department and -profession mentorship). My mentor and I did not focus so much on the details of the organisation and job, except when I had a specific question; rather we focused on my reason for being there at all, where I saw my career and life going, and how I might use my current role to get there. A warm, talented, and inspiring person, she and I were able to focus on my interests in feminism, solution-focused approaches, and our shared values. The experience was transformational and really taught me the benefit of mentorship and how it can co-exist with supervision in the career of a health and social care professional. I have since gone on to mentor others myself.

Coaching

'**Coaching**' is another form of one-to-one professional development support (although we will discuss its use in groups later). Coaching tends to be time-limited and focused on developing a particular skill set. It could also be used when moving through a challenge, and/or working towards a particular professional goal.

There is a lack of agreement among coaching professionals about an exact definition, but there are some agreed characteristics of coaching, namely that it:

- focuses on improving performance
- includes organisational and individual goals
- uses solution-focused techniques
- assists professionals to reframe challenges, and
- is a skilled activity which should be delivered by people with specific training (Chartered Institute of Personnel Development, 2020).

Specific training is required because coaching is recognised as an emergent profession in its own right. Over the last 25 years, the International Coaching Federation (ICF) has grown to provide governance, training, and support for the coaching community (ICF, 2021). A coach may have experience in your own profession, but it is not always necessary as they can still support the coachee without this domain-specific knowledge. Our Editor's **Reflective Story (Box 1.4)** in this section shares an experience of coaching, before we move on to discuss the purpose and function of supervision.

BOX 1.4

Editor's Reflective Story: Experience of coaching

After 24 years working for various public sector organisations, I (Steph) decided I wanted to become self-employed so I could pursue specific projects of interest (like making time to write this book!). I have learned from experience that when I face periods of transition, whether personal and/or professional, I benefit from additional scaffolding to help me manage periods of substantial change.

As a complete novice to life as a business owner, I built a team around me for professional and personal development support. I have one formal, qualified coach who helps me articulate my business offer based on my personal and professional values, and supporting my business planning efforts. I have another task-based informal coach (who works with me as my accountant) to teach me the skill set I need to set up the business, from tax and financial perspectives. And I have peers who I meet with for group supervision. As I settled into life running my own business, I noticed old, unhelpful behaviours and thoughts re-emerging. I know from experience that these can undermine my efforts and abilities. So, I also chose to work with a counsellor, recognising the expertise they bring to my team.

FUNCTIONS OF SUPERVISION

The functions of supervision are formed largely around **educational**, **administrative**, and **supportive needs**, with the focus on the supervisee. These functions can overlap, meaning that flexibility is needed from both the supervisor and supervisee. For example, a supervisee wanting to debrief following a complex and challenging experience is not only tapping into the supportive function of supervision (e.g. debriefing, discussing stress-management and coping skills), but also tapping into the educational functions (e.g. identifying further professional development or education needs that have become apparent from that situation).

Supervision offers a range of benefits. Firstly, it can be seen as a safety mechanism for the public and professionals. In many organisations it is the less experienced people who undertake most of the operational work, with more experienced people assuming managerial or strategic positions, becoming further away from the day-to-day demands and risk (Leary, 2018). Effective supervision may partly mitigate some of this risk, as knowledge is shared and best practices are supported through formalised interactions between more and less experienced people.

Supervision offers a range of benefits for professionals too. It helps people feel supported in their work, offers a platform to debrief, discuss and develop coping skills and stress-management strategies, and improves skills and knowledge to perform competently (Martin and Snowdon, 2020).

The benefits of supervision to organisations are also recognised. For example, supervision has a positive effect on staff recruitment and retention, intent-to-stay in a role, job satisfaction, quality of life, and burnout and absenteeism (Martin et al., 2019). Chapter 9 of this book will explore supervision from managerial and strategic perspectives as we seek to place the development of supervision within a broader context.

To enable supervision to function effectively, we need to create a safe space and time for people to learn and grow, and we will discuss this in the next section.

CREATING SAFE SPACES AND TIME FOR SUPERVISION

The concept of a **safe space** might feel self-explanatory, and you may be wondering if you even need to read this section. So, to help you make your decision, we invite you to read Gill's story.

> **BOX 1.5**
>
> **Reflective Story by Gill Taylor: The importance of a safe space for supervision**
>
> I have always considered my supervision as a necessary part of my professional practice and valued it to keep me on track, to help me advance my capability, and to enhance my knowledge and skills. However, within my supervisory sessions – be that peer supervision, one-to-one, or in a group – I don't ever remember lowering my professional guard. Was I so busy being professional that I forgot I was also human? Would it somehow have made me less professional to let my guard down and show my human side?

But there came a point in time that, due to experiencing depression and anxiety, I found myself in a position of vulnerability and was completely overwhelmed by the circumstances. At this point, I chose to begin supervision with an integrative psychotherapist and professional supervisor. From these sessions I was able to reflect on my previous supervision experiences and reframe my perspective of how supervision has the potential to support practice professionally and, of equal importance, personally.

For the first time in my professional occupational therapy career, I experienced what it was to be in a 'safe space' within supervision. These sessions provided the perfect environment I needed to allow myself to 'drop' the professionalism and to breathe, offload, reflect, be restored, grow, and to get my feet back on solid ground to move forward. It has taken me a long time to accept that supervision can be everything I need it to be, so I can support myself to support others.

In Gill's story, we learn that before experiencing professional supervision, Gill did not allow her "professional guard" down in previous supervision sessions. This is a concept that has been recognised within the literature, such as in a study undertaken by Sweeney et al. (2001a), where supervisees discussed their need to maintain a professional face in supervision. It may be difficult to create a safe supervisory space for several reasons, including when a supervisor serves dual professional and managerial roles, so is expected to evaluate performance, is responsible for yearly appraisals, and may write future job references. From this we could conclude that, to create a safe space, we need to be supervised by someone who is not our line manager.

While there might be some truth in that, Gill also identified that she did not let her professional guard down even in peer supervision, where there was no line management interference. From conversations we had while writing this book, it appears peer supervision is also difficult for some independent practitioners where peers feel more like business competitors. These examples suggest there are other factors beyond line manager/supervisor relationships that affect our ability to create a safe space. We will return to these ideas in detail in Chapter 4, but for now we wanted to consider how time may be another critical factor in supervision.

To illustrate the importance of making time for supervision (and mentoring), we would like to share a story by Jenniffer, an occupational therapist from Chile who investigated cross-cultural mentoring strategies to build capacity during her PhD studies through an Australian University. Jenniffer's findings from her research have been developed into the **cross-cultural model of mentoring** (García Rojas, n.d.). While related to mentoring, we think the ideas apply to supervision. To use this model involves identifying local champions and working together to build genuine partnerships that value and respect the expertise of both mentors and mentees, as well as continuously engaging in reflection that facilitates cultural awareness and sensitivity. The inner part of the model highlights one principle that pervades each step of the process: **change takes time**. Jenniffer shares her examples of the importance of time in the following **Reflective Story (Box 1.6)**.

BOX 1.6

Reflective Story by Jenniffer García Rojas: The importance of time for mentoring and supervision

Over the last four years of my PhD study, with my supervisors, we have developed a model to facilitate mentoring between occupational therapists from different cultures. Our aim is to share knowledge about successful mentoring to improve the quality of occupational therapy practice worldwide.

I am a bilingual mentor with knowledge of occupational therapy in Chile and Australia, and I have been supported by my Australian PhD supervisors (who were also mentors in the study). Together we have worked with occupational therapists from Chile (the mentees) to build capacity for evidence-based and occupation-centred practice.

Our study revealed how time played an essential role in successful mentoring, and hence we placed it at the centre of our model. Specifically, time was highlighted in four key areas:

First, goal setting takes time. Mentors' understanding of the mentees' practice developed gradually during the time spent together online. Even though mentors (who were experienced occupational therapists) used their skills to gather information about the context from the beginning of the study to facilitate goal setting, the mentors' hidden assumptions (and lots of 'Aha!' moments about how practice actually worked in Chile) emerged as mentors and mentees told each other stories about their practice in Chile and in Australia. Taking time to understand each other enabled the formulation of culturally and contextually relevant mentee goals.

Second, mentors need time to learn from and about the context. While there was a recognition that there would be some differences in occupational therapy practices between Australia and Chile, it was only through time and consistent engagement that mentors and mentees came to appreciate the nuanced differences between the contexts. For example, in Australia it may be common to use assessment tools to understand a situation and keep track of progress. But assuming that it would be similar in Chile presented difficulties, as in Chile there was limited access to assessment tools. Thus, outcomes were subjectively measured through observing, for example, if a child behaved better, cried less, or improved according to the occupational therapist's opinion. Mentors needed time and an intentional focus to learn about the context, so their guidance would be relevant for mentees.

Third, mentees and mentors need regular time together to monitor progress. Through weekly communication, the project enabled mutual capacity building: Chilean mentees implemented research knowledge and made changes in practice that they perceived were meaningful to their contexts; and the Australian mentors developed a new understanding of principles to develop cross-cultural partnerships in occupational therapy.

Finally, time and support are required to create change in practice. Finding a common ground between how mentors and mentees made changes to their practice required time. For example, a mentee could not understand why some children and families did not engage and comply with her therapy plans. Reflective practice was not common in Chile (García Rojas et al., 2017), so the mentee was guided through a reflective process over several weeks. Through this process, the mentor and mentee identified that there were different views about the importance of using a person-centred approach, and the role that intrinsic motivation and self-determination play in engaging people in therapy (D'Arrigo et al., 2019). Once these concepts were introduced and considered in context, the mentee understood the importance of shared goal setting and made progress with the child and family.

Jenniffer's story highlighted the importance of taking the time to develop relationships and understand different contexts and being prepared to invest sufficient time and energy for meaningful changes to happen in practice. Both Jenniffer's and Gill's stories raise interesting perspectives that could have relevance for your own supervisory situation, so we invite you to consider the questions posed in **Box 1.7**.

BOX 1.7

Reflecting on the importance of time and a safe space for supervision

- What do you feel were the key ingredients to creating the 'safe space' that Gill talks about?
- What do you feel were the key ideas raised by Jenniffer?
- How does creating time and a safe supervisory space relate to your own experiences and situations?

Chapter 3 will offer a new framework for identifying the components of effective supervision which, if attended to, could support the creation of the right environment. We will also return to Gill's story to learn more about her reflections in relation to the new framework, and we invite you to keep hold of your answers to the questions in Box 1.7 so you can link and develop your own thoughts. In Chapter 4, we will also discuss other topics that impact on the creation of time and a safe supervision space, including revisiting our understanding of self-care, exploring defence mechanisms, and engaging in the concept of elegant challenge. For now, we will discuss some other practical considerations when engaging in supervision, and how frameworks and models can help us structure what we do.

SUPERVISION FRAMEWORKS

This section will give a brief overview of some of the frameworks (i.e. tools to guide your thinking), and the next section will outline models of supervision (i.e. concepts to organise your thinking), most of which originate and extend beyond the occupational therapy profession. It is by no means an exhaustive overview, and we encourage wider reading.

Supervision frameworks are useful in guiding the supervisee and supervisor. Frameworks can help by offering tools that link theories and models of supervision to practice. Often, supervision frameworks and models are used by organisations to inform supervision guidelines. Depending on your local and national context, different guidelines for supervision will apply. We encourage you to **seek out any guidelines that are relevant to your situation** and interpret the information according to the culture within your workplace. You may also wish to seek out guidelines that challenge your existing culture to influence change in supervision practices where you work.

In the United Kingdom, the Health and Care Professions Council (HCPC) commissioned a rapid review of supervision (HCPC, 2020) which outlined evidence to inform the questions in **Box 1.8**.

BOX 1.8

The Health and Care Professions Council (HCPC)'s rapid review of supervision questions (HCPC, 2020)

1. What do individuals need from a system of clinical or peer supervision, and what areas should supervision focus on?
2. What are the outcomes of effective one-to-one clinical supervision and peer supervision?
3. What are the barriers to effective one-to-one clinical and peer supervision?
4. How much supervision is appropriate?
5. Could distance one-to-one clinical or peer supervision be effective?
6. What should employers consider and focus on when offering or designing one-to-one clinical or peer supervision?
7. How should a system of supervision be implemented?
8. Is there any need to implement supervision differently for different professionals?
9. Are there circumstances in which one-to-one clinical or peer supervision is preferable to traditional models of managerial supervision?

In summary, the research identified ten **characteristics as key for effective supervision**, including

- a supervisory relationship built on trust
- a choice of supervisor
- a shared understanding of the purpose of supervision
- regular supervision based on need
- the use of supervision models, and
- training for supervisors.

Practical challenges such as lack of time, heavy workload, and a need for clarity on the purpose of supervision were recognised. An internet search for the HCPC supervision webpages will direct you to further details and resources to support supervision practices.

There are also frameworks that focus on specific aspects of supervision. The Health Workforce Australia (HWA) National Clinical Supervision Competency Resource Framework was developed in 2013 to guide student supervision, but it has been useful when applied to professional supervision as well. It documents core competencies of supervisors across multiple healthcare disciplines and there is provision for it to be used as a tool to assess the supervision competency of individuals (HWA, 2013).

Before selecting a supervision framework, we invite you to consider the critical questions in **Box 1.9** as part of helping you find something to suit your needs.

BOX 1.9

Critical questions when selecting a supervision framework

1. Are supervision frameworks (or guidance) available within my organisation?
2. Are supervision frameworks available through my national professional association or regulatory body?
3. Are there any supervision frameworks for health or related professions which could offer useful advice?
4. Are there any recommended or compulsory standards for supervision (within my organisation, locally, or nationally)?
5. Are there any supervision frameworks used for student supervision (e.g. available from a local occupational therapy education programme) that I can apply to my workplace context?
6. What are the outcomes of effective supervision that we want to see?

MODELS OF SUPERVISION

When deciding on what to include in supervision, supervision models, like frameworks, can help. Knowing what is going to be included (and excluded) helps the organisation, supervisor, and supervisee understand expectations. There are several models of supervision described in the literature, and we will share a few here. However, when considering models of supervision, we must be aware that many have been constructed, practised, and evaluated within a Western paradigm, including within cultures where less dominant voices are not always heard (Beddoe, 2015).

Proctor's Working Alliance Model (2001)

The work of Brigid Proctor has been influential and widely adopted across many health and social care professions since the 1980s. A detailed description of the complete working alliance model is beyond the scope of this book (see Proctor, 2001), but it absorbs earlier work in which Proctor (1986) described the three functions and tasks for supervision. They are framed as benefits to the supervisee rather than specific processes. **Proctor's three functions of supervision are**:

- **Formative (educational elements)** – developing skills, knowledge, and capabilities to fulfil the duties of the role and develop as a professional.
- **Normative (norms of the organisation and profession)** – adhering to policies, procedures, guidelines, protocols, etc. associated with the role, employing organisation, and/or professional body.
- **Restorative (supportive elements)** – support and guidance, coping with stress and complex work situations, emotional wellbeing of the supervisee.

Several frameworks and guidance documents cite Proctor's work, and the three functions of supervision; e.g. NHS Education Scotland (2020) has embedded the functions into their practical resource on support and supervision for allied health professionals.

Connecting Practice: A Practitioner Centred Model of Supervision (Nancarrow et al., 2014)

The Connecting Practice: A Practitioner Centred Model of Supervision was developed following an analysis of multiple supervision frameworks used by health professionals in rural and remote settings (Nancarrow et al., 2014). From the 17 supervision frameworks reviewed, **13 domains of supervision** were identified, and these are shown in **Box 1.10**.

BOX 1.10

Connecting Practice: 13 domains of supervision (Nancarrow et al., 2014)

1. Definitions
2. Purpose and function
3. Supervision models
4. Contexts
5. Content
6. Modes of engagement

7. Supervisor attributes
8. Supervisory relationships
9. Supervisor responsibilities
10. Supervisee responsibilities
11. Structures/process for supervision and support
12. Facilitators and barriers
13. Outcomes

These domains are recommended as a starting point for services wishing to set out a policy on supervision or to help guide the development of a supervision agreement (see Chapter 5). In Chapter 3, we will share with you some work we have done to synthesise these domains with the content of other frameworks and models, to distil the essence of what we believe makes supervision effective.

The Seven-Eyed Model of Supervision (Hawkins and McMahon, 2020)

This model has been developed over the last 35 years by Professor Peter Hawkins primarily for counsellors and psychotherapists, although it is used across professions including those in health and social care (see Hawkins and McMahon, 2020, for a detailed description, application, and critique of the latest version).

In short, within the context of supervision over time, rather than within every session, attention must be paid to seven different elements. Some of the elements, known as modes, focus on the presentation of self and the relationships between a supervisee, a supervisor, and the people accessing their services; some modes focus on the wider contexts in which the supervisee works.

The presentation of the seven different modes allows you to explore questions such as:

- Thinking about the person you are working with – what theories help you to understand their difficulties?
- Is there anything you wished you had done differently in your work with this person so far?
- What sort of relationship do you have with them? How are you interacting with them? How does this make you feel?
- What resources are available to you that you could utilise more?

This model has detailed descriptions of the seven modes. We would also suggest that this is not an entry-level supervision model and, if you are interested, you may need to invest time to explore the ideas.

Tandem Model of Clinical Supervision (Milne and James, 2005)

While the quality and effectiveness of any supervision arrangement is dependent on both the supervisor and the supervisee, the instrumental role played by the supervisor in 'steering' in the right direction cannot be overestimated. The Tandem Model of Clinical Supervision highlights the importance of the supervisor by positioning them as the leader (Milne and James, 2005).

In this model, the supervisor and supervisee are viewed as two cyclists on a tandem bicycle. The supervisor occupies the front seat, thereby steering the tandem, controlling the brakes, and changing gears as required. The supervisee occupies the metaphorical backseat and is depicted clearly as the follower. However, there are opportunities for the supervisee to cycle solo and go on some 'trips' in an empowered role.

The Tandem Model depicts the crucial leadership role that the supervisor needs to play, as well as emphasises the need for a collaborative partnership where both the supervisee and supervisor are well aligned on the journey of supervision (Milne and James, 2005). However, both the supervisor and supervisee have a key responsibility to steer and work together to reach their desired destination.

The Queer People of Color (QPOC) Resilience-Based Model of Supervision (Singh and Chun, 2010)

Singh and Chun (2010) drew upon a general lack of literature and their own personal histories as queer people of colour to develop a model of supervision that aims to bring together pre-existing multicultural and queer models of supervision (Gray et al., 2001; Halpert et al., 2007). They were responding to a perceived need for a model of supervision that:

• considered identification with multiple identities, such as race and sexuality (often called **intersectionality**), rather than one aspect of identity only
• focused on the role of supervisor development as a key aspect of effective supervision, and
• acknowledged the resilience that people with multiple identities, such as queer people of colour, have, and made use of it within supervision.

Singh and Chun (2010) state that the primary goal of supervision is to support supervisee development. To achieve this, they emphasise the **need for supervisor development**, as without it, supervision may not be culturally safe and affirmative. Therefore, this model focuses on how the supervisor can promote resilience (the central concept in **Figure 1.1**) through continuous self-reflection.

To apply the model, supervisors – particularly supervisors of people who identify with multiple groups and experience intersectionality – focus on self-reflection (reflect-in-action) on their own awareness of privilege and oppression, their affirmation of diversity, and their own empowerment (the three corner triangles in Figure 1.1). Specific reflective questions are provided to help structure these reflections as supervision moves across six process domains (depicted as the six inner triangles in Figure 1.1). To get you started, **Box 1.11** shares examples of self-reflection questions from the first process domain, **supervisor-focused personal development** (Singh and Chun, 2010).

Acknowledging experiences with privilege and oppression equips supervisors to engage safely in discussions about diversity with supervisees. If you found reflecting on these questions useful, Singh and Chun (2010) have many more reflection questions you could work through and use in your supervisory practice. We will also discuss this model further in Chapter 4.

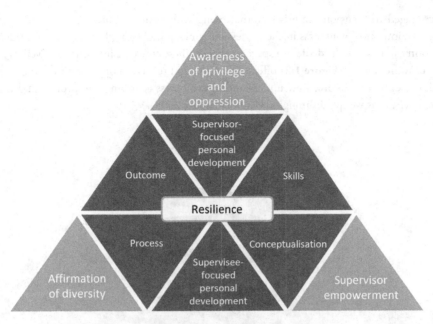

FIGURE 1.1 The Queer People of Colour (QPOC) Resilience-Based Model of Supervision (adapted from Singh and Chun, 2010)

BOX 1.11

Self-reflection questions from the Queer People of Colour (QPOC) Resilience-Based Model of Supervision (Singh and Chun, 2010)

Domain 1: Supervisor-focused personal development	Self-reflection questions
Awareness of privilege and oppression	What identities allow me to experience privilege?
Affirmation of diversity	With which aspects of diversity do I still struggle?
Supervisor empowerment	Think about a resilience experience in which I successfully challenged myself to reflect upon and learn from my shortcomings. How can I draw upon that experience to continue developing as a supervisor?

The Cyclical Model of White Awareness and its use in supervision (Ryde, 2009)

Based on her doctoral research, Judy Ryde (2009) presents the Cyclical Model of White Awareness and devotes a chapter in her book to exploring the impact of being white as a dominant identity, including in supervision. White professionals, in their capacity as a supervisor and/or supervisee, are encouraged to focus on the privilege that being white brings. Indeed, within occupational therapy, the impact of whiteness in the profession is being highlighted (e.g. Grenier, 2020), and supervision can provide the dedicated space to explore these concepts further. The Cyclical Model of White Awareness (see **Figure 1.2**) offers discussion and reflection opportunities, and has been devised as a cycle to reinforce how understanding whiteness is an ongoing process and that the learning deepens as we spiral through the model (Ryde, 2009).

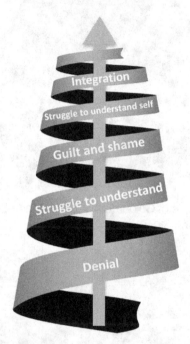

Integration

Struggle to understand self

Guilt and shame

Struggle to understand

Denial

FIGURE 1.2 Cyclical Model of White Awareness (adapted from Ryde, 2009)

Identity-Conscious Supervision Model (Brown et al., 2020)

No one is culturally neutral. We all have multiple identities that are likely to be a mix of dominant and marginalised ones. We are all products of our own upbringing, cultures, experiences, habitual ways of thinking, and values – and these collectively shape the way we think and behave, including within our supervision and supervisory relationships.

Brown et al. (2020) argue that many people leave their jobs not because of the work, but because of the environment they work within. Therefore, adopting an **Identity-Conscious Supervision Model** (Brown et al., 2020) could support recruitment and retention of a diverse workforce. The model explores concepts such as the relationship with self and others; engaging with conflict; acting with courage; managing power; and creating a strong sense of self. The authors promote the use of the model within higher education, with a particular focus on the supervisory relationships between academic staff and students; however, we feel it could be applied more widely.

In various places throughout this book, we will explore topics aligned with or included within the Identity-Conscious Supervision Model. We will consider the concepts of vulnerability, permeability, elegant challenge, courage, power dynamics, and identifying our own sphere of influence, as part of understanding the complexity of supervision. But, at this point in this book, we invite you to consider some questions that Brown et al. (2020) offer in **Box 1.12**.

BOX 1.12

Reflective questions for identity-conscious supervision (adapted from Brown et al., 2020)

- What are your dominant identities?
- How do systems of dominance and oppression show themselves in your supervision practices?
- How do systems of dominance and oppression show themselves in your workplace?
- How do systems of dominance and oppression show themselves in your wider service context?
- What are your marginalised identities?
- How can you advocate for healing in your marginalised identities?

In this section we have presented a range of models of supervision, although a quick search on the internet will no doubt find many others. Models and frameworks can help people be intentional and structured within their supervision practice. To consolidate the application of frameworks and models to supervisory practice, **Box 1.13** summarises a few additional practical tips for consideration.

BOX 1.13

Practical tips for using a framework and/or model to frame supervision

- Think about and identify components of frameworks and/or models of supervision that you feel would be of benefit to the supervisory relationship (the supervisor or supervisee could do this).
- Introduce ideas to the person if they are unfamiliar with them and discuss and agree on their use within your supervisory sessions.
- Decide how the framework and/or model will be used within the structure of the supervision documentation.
- Encourage the joint development of the supervision agenda, using the framework and/or model of supervision to guide, as appropriate.
- Agree a timescale to pilot using the framework and/or model in a specified way and then review this to ensure it is meeting everyone's needs.

What we would like to emphasise in our book is how we can responsibly engage in supervision for the benefit of all. To draw together concepts in this chapter, our final section explores inclusive supervision.

INCLUSIVE SUPERVISION

Occupational therapists are experts in analysing the person, occupation, and environmental fit for maximum occupational performance and participation (Law et al., 1996). When applying these same skills in supervision, we become aware of and responsive to people's needs, whether they relate to gender, race, religion, sexual orientation, disability, or anything else. **Recognising multiple identities exist, as we have introduced earlier in the concept of intersectionality – rather than one aspect of identity only – can also enhance our thinking and practice**. In this section on inclusive supervision, we will use the example of supervisees and supervisors who have an additional need or disability to continue our discussions, although we acknowledge intersectionality exists with multiple factors.

People we work with (or ourselves) may have a disability or additional need that is diagnosed or undiagnosed, visible or invisible, but requires consideration. For example, people may have dyslexia, depression, hearing loss, a physical difficulty or disability, a long-term condition, long COVID, or many other conditions. Applying our core occupational therapy skills to enable the maximum performance and participation of the supervisee in supervision and their work role will form a critical feature of the relationship (College of Occupational Therapists, 2015).

Every setting will be bound by different rules and regulations about disability and additional needs, and these often evolve as society refines its ideas about inclusion. It is useful to find out about any legal obligations, professional responsibilities, and organisational policies relating to inclusion, disability, accommodations, or reasonable adjustments that will impact on supervision. Ideas on reasonable adjustments and approaching this topic in supervision will be explored further in Chapter 8.

We all identify, or wish not to be identified, in certain ways. We hope to offer a space for open discussions and enhanced understanding, and to encourage this more in supervision. We particularly resonate with the idea of 'humility' rather than 'competency', which acknowledges that we are constantly learning, recognise without shame our knowledge gaps, and expect differences between and within groups (Agner et al., 2020). We will explore this further in Chapter 4, but invite you to consider **Box 1.14** and our ideas on supporting others whatever their needs.

BOX 1.14

A starting point for supporting people to share their individual needs

- Create a safe space for a conversation to discuss any needs.
- Consider approaching the conversation from an appreciative, strengths-based perspective (see Chapter 2).

- Think about how you would approach a person accessing services who needed support or advice to perform in the workplace. Are there any elements that could be applied in this situation?
- Discuss specific situations that frequently happen at work, and what could be adjusted to make the job more doable. This may feel less overwhelming than trying to look at the job as a whole.

CRITICAL COMMENTARY

Supervision is complicated. Or is it joyful, rewarding, inspiring, and affirming ... or all of the above?

Supervision, and the process of doing supervision well, is complicated and multifaceted. We can acknowledge the first point but choose to see and strive for developing supervision as a joyful, rewarding, inspiring, and affirming experience. The narrative around supervision tends to be dominated by the first point, and we would encourage you to think about how complicated supervision is (or is not) for you. Think about how we introduced supervision at the start of the book, including the editors' reflective stories. Also take some time to consider your own perceptions and experiences of supervision so far – including the importance you have placed on it versus the idea that it is something that can be dropped when life gets busy.

In this chapter we have presented frameworks and models and have explored their use to aid effective supervision. In contrast, it could be argued that frameworks and models are restrictive, inhibit creativity, and are based within dominant cultures, which fuels power dynamics. For example, consider the response if your supervisee arrives at their first session asking which supervision model you prefer – how does this make you feel if this is something you haven't thought about, and what impact does this have on your first impressions as you are forming your working relationship?

Throughout this book, we will explore several 'complicating' factors that need to be negotiated and addressed as part of making supervision effective. These include the relational aspects of supervision; the power dynamics from role, culture, and individual power (Ryde, 2009); and the need for strategic support within organisations. We acknowledge that the deeper we delve into supervision, the more complicated it may appear. While not minimising complexity, we are attempting to explore these challenges in a practical way so that the effort we put into supervision is well placed. With supervision being a public and professional safety mechanism, it makes investing in this valuable resource essential.

SUMMARY

In this introductory chapter, we have outlined our way of addressing inclusivity in this book. We have explored the definitions of some of the key terms used within this text including supervision, managerial supervision, mentoring, and coaching. We have outlined the purpose and function of supervision and considered how to create time and a safe space for important conversations. Finally, we presented a brief overview of some of the frameworks and models for supervision and how they can be helpful in framing inclusive supervisory practices.

Before heading into Chapter 2, where we explore some of the concepts that underpin supervision, we invite you to identify the topics in this chapter where you would like to deepen your own understanding and identify sources, including specific references in the list at the end of this chapter, which will help.

REFERENCES

Agner, J., Barile, J.P., Chandler, S.M., and Berry, M. (2020) 'Innovation in child welfare: factors affecting adoption of empirically supported interventions', *Children and Youth Services Review*, 119, pp. 1–10. doi:10.1016/j.childyouth.2020.105580.

American Occupational Therapy Association (1981) 'Guide for supervision of occupational therapy personnel', *American Journal of Occupational Therapy*, 35(12), pp. 815–816. doi:10.5014/ajot.35.12.815.

Beddoe, L. (2015) 'Supervision and developing the profession: one supervision or many?', *China Journal of Social Work*, 8(2), pp. 150–163. doi:10.1080/17525098.2015.1039173.

Brown, R., Desai, S., and Elliott, C. (2020) *Identity-conscious supervision in student affairs: building relationships and transforming systems*. Abingdon: Routledge.

Chartered Institute of Personnel Development (2020) *Coaching and mentoring factsheet*. Available at: www.cipd.co.uk/knowledge/fundamentals/people/development/coaching-mentoring-factsheet (Accessed: 8 May 2021).

College of Occupational Therapists (1990) *Statement on supervision in occupational therapy*. London: College of Occupational Therapists.

College of Occupational Therapists (2015) *Code of ethics and professional conduct*. London: College of Occupational Therapists.

D'Arrigo, R., Copley, J.A., Poulsen, A.A., and Ziviani, J. (2019) 'Parent engagement and disengagement in paediatric settings: an occupational therapy perspective', *Disability and Rehabilitation*, 42(20), pp. 2882–2893. doi:10.1080/09638288.2019.1574913.

Davys, A., Fouché, C., and Beddoe, L. (2021) 'Mapping effective interprofessional supervision practice', *The Clinical Supervisor*, 40(2), pp. 179–199. doi:10.1080/07325223.2021.1929639.

Fitzpatrick, S., Smith, M., and Wilding, C. (2012) 'Quality allied health clinical supervision policy in Australia: a literature review', *Australian Health Review*, 36(4), pp. 461–465. doi:10.1071/AH11053.

Gadomska-Lila, K. (2020) 'Effectiveness of reverse mentoring in creating intergenerational relationships', *Journal of Organizational Change Management*, 33(7), pp. 1313–1328.

García Rojas, J. (n.d.) A cross cultural partnership approach to developing evidence-based practice and research capacity amongst Chilean occupational therapists. PhD thesis. University of Queensland.

García Rojas, J., Copley, J., Turpin, M., and Peña Jeldes, N. (2017) 'Práctica basada en evidencia en el área pediátrica en Chile, un desafío pendiente [Evidence-based practice in paediatric settings in Chile, an imminent challenge]', *Revista Chilena de Terapia Ocupacional*, 17(2), pp. 57–68. doi:10.5354/0719-5346.2018.48086.

Gray, L.A., Ladany, N., Walker, J.A., and Ancis, J.R. (2001) 'Psychotherapy trainees' experience of counterproductive events in supervision', *Journal of Counseling Psychology*, 48(4), pp. 371–383. doi:10.1037/0022-0167.48.4.371.

Grenier, M.-L. (2020) 'Cultural competency and the reproduction of white supremacy in occupational therapy education', *Health Education Journal*, 79(6), pp. 633–644. doi:10.1177/0017896920902515.

Halpert, S.C., Reinhardt, B., and Toohey, M.J. (2007) 'Affirmative clinical supervision', in Bieschke, K.J., Perez, R.M., and DeBord, K.A. (eds) *Handbook of Counseling and Psychotherapy with Lesbian, Gay,*

Bisexual, and Transgender Clients. Washington, DC: American Psychological Association, pp. 341–358. doi:10.1037/11482-014.

Hawkins, P. and McMahon, A. (2020) *Supervision in the helping professions*. 5th edn. London: McGraw Hill/ Open University Press.

Health and Care Professions Council (2020) *The characteristics of effective supervision*. London: Health and Care Professions Council. Available at: www.hcpc-uk.org/resources/reports/2019/effective-clinical-and-peer-supervision-report/ (Accessed: 8 May 2021).

Health Education England (2020) *Workplace supervision for advanced clinical practice: an integrated multi-professional approach for practitioner development*. Available at: www.hee.nhs.uk/our-work/advanced-practice/reports-publications/workplace-supervision-advanced-clinical-practice (Accessed: 31 May 2021).

Health Workforce Australia (2013) *National clinical supervision competency resource – validation edition*. Available at: www.clinedaus.org.au/files/resources/hwa_national_clinical_supervision_competency_resource_ve_201305_2.pdf (Accessed: 11 November 2020).

International Coaching Federation (2021) *The International Coaching Federation ecosystem explained*. Available at: https://coachingfederation.org/about/the-icf-ecosystem (Accessed: 5 May 2021).

Kadushin, A. (1968) 'Games people play in supervision', *Social Work*, 13(3), pp. 23–32. doi:10.1093/sw/13.3.23.

Law, M., Cooper, B., Strong, S., Stewart, D., Rigby, P., and Letts, L. (1996) 'The Person–Environment–Occupation Model: a transactive approach to occupational performance', *Canadian Journal of Occupational Therapy*, 63(1), pp. 9–23. doi:10.1177/000841749606300103.

Leary, A. (2018) *James Reason lecture: patient safety congress*. Available at: www.youtube.com/watch?v=4sqlyvKvFlI (Accessed: 8 November 2021).

Martin, P., Copley, J., and Tyack, Z. (2014) 'Twelve tips for effective clinical supervision based on a narrative literature review and expert opinion', *Medical Teacher*, 36(3), pp. 201–207. doi:10.3109/0142159X.2013.852166.

Martin, P., Lizarondo, L., Kumar, S., and Snowdon, D. (2019) 'Impact of clinical supervision of health professionals on organizational outcomes: a mixed methods systematic review protocol', *JBI Database of Systematic Reviews and Implementation Reports*, 18(1), pp. 115–120. doi:10.11124/JBISRIR-D-19-00017.

Martin, P. and Snowdon, D. (2020) 'Can clinical supervision bolster clinical skills and well-being through challenging times?', *Journal of Advanced Nursing*, 76(11), pp. 2781–2782. doi:10.1111/jan.14483.

Milne, D. and James, I. (2005) 'Clinical supervision: ten tests of the tandem model', *Clinical Psychology Forum*, 151, pp. 6–10.

Nancarrow, S.A., Wade, R., Moran, M., Coyle, J., Young, J., and Boxall, D. (2014) 'Connecting practice: a practitioner centred model of supervision', *Clinical Governance: An International Journal*, 19(3), pp. 235–253. doi:10.1108/CGIJ-03-2014-0010.

National Health Service Education for Scotland (2020) *Support and supervision for allied health professionals*. Available at: https://learn.nes.nhs.scot/29153/allied-health-professions-ahp-learning-site/supporting-the-wellbeing-and-mental-health-of-yourself-your-team-and-others/support-and-supervision-for-allied-health-professionals-a-practical-resource-for-ahps (Accessed: 8 March 2021).

Occupational Therapy Australia (2019) *Professional supervision framework*. Melbourne: Occupational Therapy Australia. Available at: https://otaus.com.au/publicassets/2e35a9f6-b890-e911-a2c3-9b7af2531dd2/ProfessionalSupervisionFramework2019.pdf (Accessed: 13 October 2021).

Oshinkale, Y. (2019) *Definition of mentorship: what is a mentor and do you need one?* Available at: www.wes.org/advisor-blog/definition-of-mentorship. (Accessed: 13 October 2021).

Proctor, B., Marken, M., and Payne, M. (1986). 'Supervision: a cooperative exercise in accountability', in Marken, M., and Payne, M. (eds) *Enabling and ensuring: supervision in practice*. Leicester: National Youth Bureau, pp. 21–34.

Proctor, B. (2001) 'Training for the supervision alliance attitude, skills and intention', in Cutcliffe, J.R., Butterworth, T., and Proctor, B. (eds) *Fundamental themes in clinical supervision*. London: Routledge, pp. 25–46.

Royal College of Occupational Therapists (2021) *Professional standards for occupational therapy practice, conduct and ethics*. Available at: https://www.rcot.co.uk/publications/professional-standards-occupational-therapy-practice-conduct-and-ethics (Accessed: 8 May 2021).

Ryde, J. (2009) *Being white in the helping professions: developing effective intercultural awareness*. London: Jessica Kingsley Publishers.

Singh, A. and Chun, K.Y.S. (2010) '"From the margins to the center": moving towards a resilience-based model of supervision for queer people of color supervisors', *Training and Education in Professional Psychology*, 4(1), pp. 36–46. doi:10.1037/a0017373.

Snowdon, D.A. (2018) 'Clinical supervision of allied health professionals'. PhD thesis. La Trobe University.

Snowdon, D.A., Hau, R., Leggat, S.G., and Taylor, N.F. (2016) 'Does clinical supervision of health professionals improve patient safety? A systematic review and meta-analysis', *International Journal for Quality in Health Care*, 28(4), pp. 447–455. doi:10.1093/intqhc/mzw059.

Snowdon, D.A., Leggat, S.G., and Taylor, N.F. (2017) 'Does clinical supervision of healthcare professionals improve effectiveness of care and patient experience? A systematic review', *BMC Health Service Research*, 17, pp. 1–11. doi:10.1186/s12913-017-2739-5.

Sweeney, G., Webley, P., and Treacher, A. (2001a) 'Supervision in occupational therapy, part 1: the supervisor's anxieties', *British Journal of Occupational Therapy*, 64(7), pp. 337–345. doi:10.1177/030802260106400704.

Sweeney, G., Webley, P., and Treacher, A. (2001b) 'Supervision in occupational therapy, part 2: the supervisee's dilemma', *British Journal of Occupational Therapy*, 64(8), pp. 380–386. doi:10.1177/F030802260106400802.

Sweeney, G., Webley, P., and Treacher, A. (2001c) 'Supervision in occupational therapy, part 3: accommodating the supervisor and the supervisee', *British Journal of Occupational Therapy*, 64(9), pp. 426–431. doi:10.1177/030802260106400902.

Victorian Government (2019) *Victorian allied health clinical supervision framework*. Melbourne: Victorian Government. Available at: www2.health.vic.gov.au/health-workforce/allied-health-workforce/clinical-supervision-framework (Accessed: 18 August 2021).

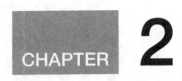

CHAPTER 2

Concepts that help us do supervision well

Karina Dancza, Stephanie Tempest, Joanne M. Baird, and Anita Volkert

With contributions from Madiha Sajid and Debbie Kramer-Roy

CHAPTER INTENTIONS

In this chapter, we invite you to:

- Apply the concepts of mindsets, motivation, and self-determination to the supervisory process
- Examine the use of appreciative, strengths-based approaches within the supervision context
- Explore selected learning and teaching principles to embed into supervision
- Reflect on professional ethics within supervision
- Identify your own learning actions to develop yourself as an effective supervisor and supervisee.

CHAPTER HIGHLIGHTS

- Mindsets, motivation, and self-determination
- Appreciative, strengths-based approaches
- Learning and teaching principles
- Professional ethical considerations
- Critical commentary: Recipes for success in supervision … if only it was that simple!

DOI: 10.4324/9781003092544-2

CHAPTER RESOURCES

Figures

- Figure 2.1 Growth and fixed mindsets continuum
- Figure 2.2 Motivation continuum
- Figure 2.3 Self-Determination Theory
- Figure 2.4 Supervision needs for career stages
- Figure 2.5 Approaches to supervision based on experience level
- Figure 2.6 Levels of practice and the Career Development Framework
- Figure 2.7 Cognitive Apprenticeship Framework
- Figure 2.8 The Professional Learning through Useful Support (PLUS) Framework for Supervision

Boxes

- Box 2.1 Illustrative example of growth and fixed mindsets
- Box 2.2 Reflective questions to help you explore your own mindset
- Box 2.3 Examples of strengths-based questions for supervision
- Box 2.4 Components of Gibbs' Model of Refection
- Box 2.5 Example questions from Rolfe's Model of Reflection
- Box 2.6 Reflective Story by Madiha Sajid and Debbie Kramer-Roy: Developing leadership skills through reflection in supervision as part of an action research project
- Box 2.7 Ethical expectations in supervision
- Box 2.8 Illustrative example of where liability could be a concern
- Box 2.9 Illustrative example of where confidentiality could be a concern
- Box 2.10 Illustrative example of where dual relationships could be a concern
- Box 2.11 Best-practice tenets for navigating complicated situations

MINDSETS, MOTIVATION, AND SELF-DETERMINATION

In Chapter 1 we explored some definitions of supervision and existing models and frameworks that help guide supervision in a broad sense. In this chapter we offer some concepts that we already know and use in our practice and explore their relevance to supervision. First, we will cover three interrelated concepts – namely growth mindset, motivation, and self-determination. Many of these concepts come from the field of psychology and have gained prominence in the education of both children and adults. We acknowledge that the translation of these concepts into supervision requires further research but feel they can offer interesting perspectives.

Growth and fixed mindsets

Carol Dweck's (2006) research over the last 30 years on effort and success suggests that people can be placed on a continuum between growth and fixed mindsets **(Figure 2.1)**, and this will influence a person's work performance and motivation. In supervision, different strategies and techniques may be required depending on how a person sees themselves along this continuum.

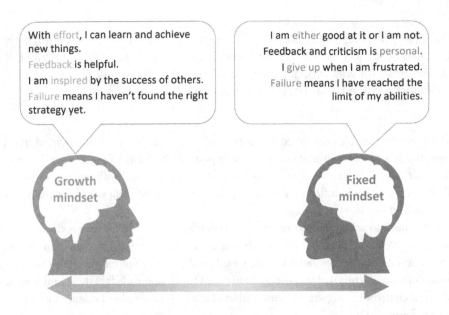

FIGURE 2.1 Growth and fixed mindsets continuum (adapted from Dweck, 2006)

Someone who is **fixed in their mindset** tends to see their talents and skills as something they were born with that cannot be changed. They will likely work to what they see is their capacity but not push themselves further, choosing easier tasks that require minimal effort. When they experience failure, it is seen as permanent, so there is no need to learn from it and try again. Feedback can also be a challenge as it is potentially seen as a personal attack (Dweck, 2006).

Someone with a **growth mindset** sees that learning does not stop at formal education. They tend to see failure as an opportunity to learn something new and improve their performance. They are open to developing themselves and see that practice and feedback are ways to do this. Obstacles or challenges are viewed as a chance to experiment with different ways of working (Dweck, 2006). To help make the difference between fixed and growth mindsets clear, we offer the following illustrative example **(Box 2.1)**.

BOX 2.1

Illustrative example of growth and fixed mindsets

Marcus is a supervisor, and he has been told by his supervisee (Simon) that he delivers feedback in quite a blunt and direct manner, which can be uncomfortable. While being a bit shocked by Simon's feedback, Marcus adopts a growth mindset and believes that he can change and develop in his ability to offer constructive feedback in supervision. Marcus sees it as a learning opportunity and seeks further feedback and advice from his own supervisor and looks for professional development opportunities to extend his knowledge.

In contrast, if Marcus adopted a fixed mindset following Simon's feedback, he may have believed that Simon simply does not 'get his style'. Marcus could hold the view that he was brought up to state bluntly how things are, and people should just get used to it. Thus, Marcus sees no need to change.

The previous example is designed to illustrate what we mean by growth and fixed mindsets. However, this is a rather simplistic perspective of a person's thinking. In practice, as illustrated in Figure 2.1, it is more helpful to view the concepts of growth and fixed mindsets as a continuum. It is likely that we all are in different places on the continuum at different times, depending on the situation we find ourselves in.

We also need to acknowledge that there are other factors beyond our perception of our own intelligence that could explain our behaviours and their outcomes. Critics of the growth mindset concept point out that it does not adequately explain the role of aptitude and fails to recognise the impact of wider factors such as poverty. However, Dweck acknowledges these limitations, and further research investigating the implementation of the growth mindset evidence into practice is underway (Severs, 2020).

Nonetheless, it could be helpful to explore your response to challenge and learning and that of your supervisor/supervisee, through the lens of the growth mindset concept. **Box 2.2** offers some reflective questions to consider.

BOX 2.2

Reflective questions to help you explore your own mindset

- Is there someone you know (a colleague, supervisor, supervisee, or friend) who displays more of a fixed mindset – someone who avoids risks, who does not admit mistakes, who cannot cope, or who gets defensive after setbacks? Do you understand that person better now? At the same time, what other factors could be affecting their ability to admit mistakes?
- Is there someone you know who displays more of a growth mindset – tries different strategies when something does not work, is keen to learn more, and works their way through obstacles? What other characteristics do they have, and what else do you know about them that might affect their ability to grow?
- Think about a time during the past month when you were faced with a work, academic, social, or personal challenge. Think about how you faced that challenge – with a growth or a fixed mindset?
  o How do you know?
  o If you faced the challenge with a fixed mindset, how might you have approached it differently?
  o What underlying habits and behaviours might have influenced your approach?

o   Do you think that there have been times in your life when it has been easier, or harder, to adopt a growth mindset?

o   What does this tell you about what might need to be in place in your environment to help you adopt a growth mindset?

Motivation

To support someone's development through supervision it can be helpful to understand something about why they do what they do. Are they motivated by such things as recognition, career progression, or something external to themselves? Or are they driven by inner desire for fulfilment or a sense of curiosity, which comes from within themselves? You may like to reflect on your own motivations and how they have influenced your career choices to date. Levels of motivation range from amotivation to extrinsic (external) motivation through to intrinsic (internal) motivation (Ziviani and Poulsen, 2015; **Figure 2.2**).

Amotivation is when someone has no will or desire to do something, so nothing is likely to happen. **Extrinsic motivation** is when someone will do something because there is an external pressure to act (reward or punishment), such as money, status, power, or to avoid being fired from a job. Thus, something will happen when the right incentive or disincentive is provided. **Intrinsic motivation** is when someone will do something because they want to. Through doing the thing, it provides a sense of achievement, joy, being challenged, or learning something new.

The reason Figure 2.2 is illustrated as a gauge is because **typically people's motivation will change depending on the situation**, rather than being fixed at one of the levels. For example, a person may be intrinsically motivated to learn about supervision practice (such as reading this book) as they gain a sense of satisfaction from improving the way they do it (intrinsic motivation). Or, a person may be required to undertake supervision (as a supervisor

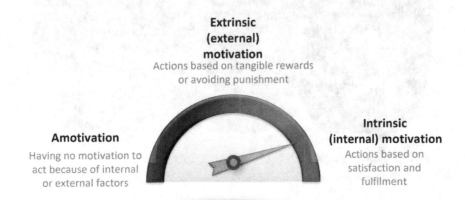

FIGURE 2.2 Motivation continuum (adapted from Ziviani and Poulsen, 2015)

or supervisee) because it is expected as part of their job and is an unavoidable task (extrinsic motivation). You may also fall somewhere between the two, as some supervisory tasks may be an essential part of your job, while you also are interested in developing your skills in supervision, so choose to do some additional learning.

Self-Determination Theory

Another example of a motivational theory applied within occupational therapy has been through the work of Anne Poulsen, Jenny Ziviani, and Monica Cuskelly (2015) and their account of Self-Determination Theory (Ryan and Deci, 2000). **Self-Determination Theory helps us understand key motivational processes that influence how someone does something**. By understanding these processes it is possible to collaboratively adjust factors within the person, occupation, and environment interplay to influence someone's actions.

Within Self-Determination Theory there are three motivational processes: **autonomy, relatedness, and competence** (Ryan and Deci, 2000). Attending to each of these psychological needs enhances the likelihood of a person moving towards an intrinsically motivated state, and all three could be considered from the perspective of the supervisor and the supervisee. **Figure 2.3** illustrates how the three motivational processes could look in supervision. Further reading is recommended to appreciate the details of this theory.

Understanding a little about mindsets, motivation, and self-determination can potentially offer insights into your relationships within supervision. In the next section we will explore how we can approach supervision from an appreciative, strengths-based perspective.

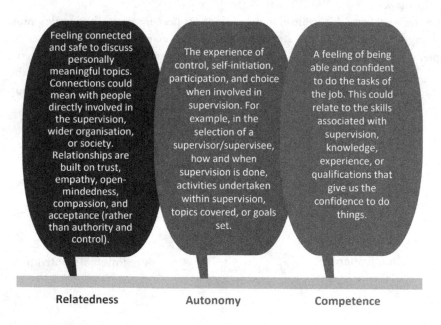

Feeling connected and safe to discuss personally meaningful topics. Connections could mean with people directly involved in the supervision, wider organisation, or society. Relationships are built on trust, empathy, open-mindedness, compassion, and acceptance (rather than authority and control).

The experience of control, self-initiation, participation, and choice when involved in supervision. For example, in the selection of a supervisor/supervisee, how and when supervision is done, activities undertaken within supervision, topics covered, or goals set.

A feeling of being able and confident to do the tasks of the job. This could relate to the skills associated with supervision, knowledge, experience, or qualifications that give us the confidence to do things.

Relatedness   **Autonomy**   **Competence**

FIGURE 2.3 Self-Determination Theory (adapted from Poulsen et al., 2015)

APPRECIATIVE, STRENGTHS-BASED APPROACHES

Appreciative, strengths-based approaches can include solution-focused and appreciative perspectives, among others. The philosophy of appreciative, strengths-based approaches is based on this premise: **if it works, do more of it; if it does not work, do something different**. They tend to be present- and future-focused rather than dwelling on past experiences (Bannink, 2007). These approaches may be particularly helpful if a challenging situation needs to be turned around quickly, or if a supervisory relationship has descended into an experience that all parties dread.

Appreciative, strengths-based approaches take a positive view of people, so it is fundamental that the supervisor comes from a perspective that **people are resourceful, able, and have the capability to change their situation**. This may take a shift in mindset, as we are often faced with deficit-led (i.e. problem-focused) perspectives. Using an appreciative, strengths-based view, small changes can lead to bigger changes. Creating space for people to explore their own solutions is also an important aspect. Other key points include that feedback is not considered failure; people will invest in the solutions they create for themselves; small successes can be built upon; and compliments, acknowledgement, and affirmation help (de Shazer et al., 2021).

In contrast to a problem-solving approach that begins with what is going wrong, appreciative, strengths-based approaches embrace **positive framing** – that is, identifying what you are doing well, what you want to do more of, and then directing your actions towards this outcome (Stavros et al., 2018). As a supervisor approaching a session from an appreciative, strengths-based perspective, you may draw from a range of question types to help the supervisee move closer to their goals. **Box 2.3** offers a starting point, and we will be building on these ideas throughout the book.

BOX 2.3

Examples of strengths-based questions for supervision

Probing questions

Invites a supervisee to expand and examine the situation in greater depth.

- Tell me about the situation, what happened next?
- Can you tell me more about that?
- What else was happening?

Explorative

Opens new ideas and encourages consideration of different perspectives.

- What if [something was different]?
- What might [someone else] say about the situation?
- What might happen if things were much better, what would that look like?

Affective

Invites a supervisee to share their feelings about a situation.

- How do you feel about what happened?
- What are you feeling about it right now?

Reflective

Encourages thinking about what is going well and what can be improved.

- What did you find interesting or surprising about the situation?
- What did you do well?
- What would you like to do differently?

Analytical

Prompts a supervisee to consider what is influencing the situation, what could be potential causes, or the pros and cons of the situation.

- What do you think was happening here?
- What is your overall view of this situation?

Clarifying

Helps to check understanding of the information presented.

- Can you tell me more about that?
- Can you please explain a bit more to me about [a certain aspect]?
- Is what you mean … [paraphrase or summarise the concept]?

Creating connections

Encourages a supervisee to make links between the situation and other situations or the broader context.

- What do you think might be the impact or consequence of doing/not doing this?
- How might this link with what you will do next?

Scaling

Helps the supervisee visualise where they are and what it might look like if they were to progress towards their goal. The intention is not necessarily to focus on the numbers (e.g. on a scale of 1–10 where 1 is not at all and 10 is all achieved), but to think about why they placed themselves at a point on the scale.

- What tells you that you are at that point on the scale?
- Where would someone else place you on that scale?
- If you were to move one point up, what would that look like?
- At what point would you consider it to be good enough?

Capabilities

Capability questions are designed to help the supervisee recognise the positives of the situation and the successful strategies they already have.

- How did you manage to do that?
- How might you use that knowledge in another area?
- What have you done in the past that might help now?
- How did you decide that was a good idea?

Outcomes

Outcome questions help the supervisee to plan of what they will do next. This attempts to bridge the supervision discussions with behavioural changes.

- What would be the three things you will do differently?
- When will you start?
- From the list of ideas we generated, what few things seem doable in the next week?
- What will you need to make this happen?
- Is there any support I can give?

LEARNING AND TEACHING PRINCIPLES

As supervisors we take on a range of roles to support learning, including fieldwork or placement supervisor, academic, and research positions, facilitating learning with people who access services, and developing a team. These roles use learning and teaching principles. As supervision offers a platform for learning, including stimulating the development of professional reasoning (Schell, 2018), we will introduce a few of these learning and teaching principles next.

Novice to expert and the different requirements for supervision

Dreyfus and Dreyfus (1980) proposed a novice-to-expert continuum of five stages in the development of skills or competencies. Within this continuum, the **learner moves though the stages of novice to advanced beginner, competent, proficient, and – finally – expert**. Benner (1984) linked this idea to clinical competence in the nursing profession, and later Craik and McKay (2003) proposed this model to identify the characteristics of expert-level consultant occupational therapists in the United Kingdom.

Understanding these different stages, and therefore the changing needs of supervisees, allows us to tailor supervision effectively. For example, when we are starting out in a career as an occupational therapist, we will have different goals, aims, and objectives, and these will change as we gain experience and expertise. This is explained further in **Figure 2.4**. Our response to supervision will also change as we gain experience and our emotional responses evolve. Being aware of these factors allows both the supervisor and the supervisee to consider which approaches might be the most effective **(Figure 2.5)**.

The stage we are at in our career has also been described in a range of ways and is constantly being refined within occupational therapy. To provide a common language for these career stages, one framework that we (Steph and Karina) have led the development and implementation of is the **Royal College of Occupational Therapists Career Development Framework** (RCOT, 2021). This framework is for occupational therapy personnel including support workers, at any

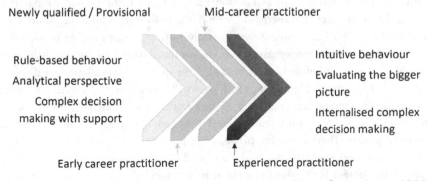

Newly qualified / Provisional   Mid-career practitioner

Rule-based behaviour
Analytical perspective
Complex decision
making with support

Intuitive behaviour
Evaluating the bigger picture
Internalised complex decision making

Early career practitioner   Experienced practitioner

FIGURE 2.4 Supervision needs for career stages (adapted from Stoltenberg, 1998)

Level of practitioner	Needs supervision to	Type of supervision needed
Newly qualified / Provisional / Transitional practitioner	• Increase understanding and skills	• Information provision • Modelling of needed behaviours and skills
Early career practitioner	• Develop specific skills to respond to novel situations	• Opportunities for practice and reflection • Structure for supervision sessions
Mid-career practitioner	• Reflect on practices • Develop complex skills • Increase innovation	• Ability to self-structure supervision sessions • Focus on challenging situations
Experienced practitioner	• Obtain varied perspectives and information	• Exposure to additional models, methods, and techniques

FIGURE 2.5 Approaches to supervision based on experience level (adapted from Swalwell and Harvey, 2017)

career stage, to help them identify where they are in relation to the four pillars of practice (common to any role), namely:

- professional practice
- facilitation of learning
- leadership, and
- evidence, research, and development.

Each of the four pillars has nine career levels. The intention is for occupational therapists to map themselves into the pillars and levels to identify areas of strength and areas for further learning and development within each pillar.

Continuing the evolution, Professor Alison Leary (2021) in the United Kingdom sought to define the levels of practice (experience) within the healthcare workforce. With a data set of approximately 45,000 healthcare workers (mainly nurses) it was possible to identify seven different levels of practice for the regulated and non-regulated workforce, conceptualised as: supportive, assistive, novice, intermediate, enhanced, advanced, and consultant. To illustrate this development, we have created **Figure 2.6**, which shows RCOT's nine career levels and four pillars of practice alongside the practice levels from Alison's work. In acknowledgement of the strategic workforce, we chose to add another practice level – director – to capture national and international strategic leaders. There is overlap between the practice and career levels, acknowledging there is a range of experience, expertise, and responsibilities in different roles.

Career development is not always linear or hierarchical. As you can see in Figure 2.6, the practice levels (e.g. novice, intermediate, enhanced) are not a direct match to the career levels (i.e. 1–9). Similarly, you can be at different career and practice levels on each pillar (i.e. professional

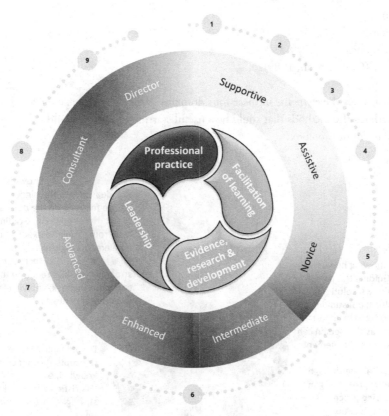

FIGURE 2.6 Levels of practice and the Career Development Framework (adapted from Leary, 2021; RCOT, 2021)

practice; facilitation of learning; leadership; and evidence, research, and development), depending on the requirements of your job and your experience. For example, an occupational therapy technician may be part of the assistive workforce, and we could assume a certain level of supervisory input may be needed. However, if that occupational therapy technician has worked in a wheelchair service for over ten years, and has crafted specialist knowledge and skills, their supervisory needs will be very different from a novice occupational therapist. Another example is when an occupational therapist moves between sectors. An enhanced, advanced, or even consultant practitioner moving into an academic role will experience new challenges and may feel more like a novice in this unfamiliar environment, as the demands in the facilitation of learning pillar intensify. Regardless of career or practice level, there is a range of ways to support learning and development, and we will explore the Cognitive Apprenticeship Framework next.

Cognitive Apprenticeship Framework

The Cognitive Apprenticeship Framework suggests four characteristics of ideal learning environments:

- content
- sequencing
- methods, and
- sociology (Collins et al., 1989).

Figure 2.7 outlines the elements in these four domains. While all aspects are related to supervision, it is perhaps the methods that could be a useful starting point to expand the teaching techniques we have in our toolbox.

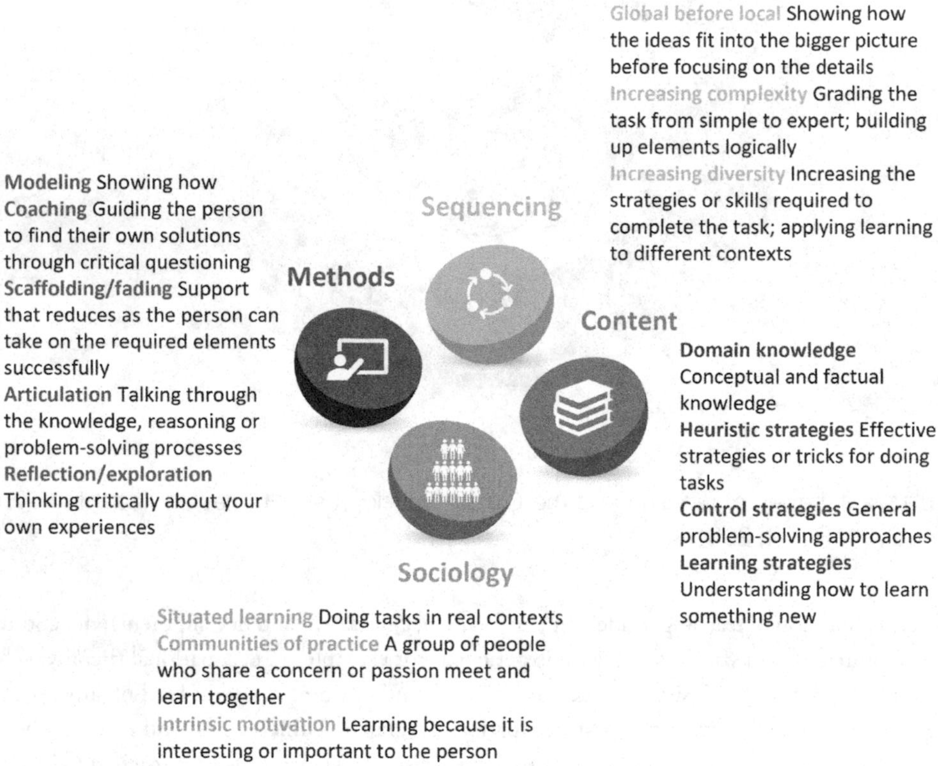

Global before local Showing how the ideas fit into the bigger picture before focusing on the details
Increasing complexity Grading the task from simple to expert; building up elements logically
Increasing diversity Increasing the strategies or skills required to complete the task; applying learning to different contexts

Modeling Showing how
Coaching Guiding the person to find their own solutions through critical questioning
Scaffolding/fading Support that reduces as the person can take on the required elements successfully
Articulation Talking through the knowledge, reasoning or problem-solving processes
Reflection/exploration Thinking critically about your own experiences

Sequencing

Methods

Content

Domain knowledge
Conceptual and factual knowledge
Heuristic strategies Effective strategies or tricks for doing tasks
Control strategies General problem-solving approaches
Learning strategies Understanding how to learn something new

Sociology

Situated learning Doing tasks in real contexts
Communities of practice A group of people who share a concern or passion meet and learn together
Intrinsic motivation Learning because it is interesting or important to the person

FIGURE 2.7 Cognitive Apprenticeship Framework (adapted from Collins et al., 1989; Schell, 2018)

The Context-Based Teaching Model for Professional Reasoning

The role of the teacher is to guide, co-create, collaborate, and enable a learner to find and interpret meaning in something (Schell, 2018). To help people who are facilitating professional reasoning in others, such as through supervision, Schell developed the Context-Based Teaching Model for Professional Reasoning. This model consolidates a range of ideas, including the Cognitive Apprenticeship Framework. It places the learner as the central focus and the teacher as someone who contextualises learning opportunities that promote professional reasoning. It does this via four main areas which are presented in a circle, indicating that you can enter at any point and move around the areas until higher levels of learning or greater independence are achieved (Schell, 2018). A brief review of the elements includes:

- **Shared experiences – authentic contexts**. Learning opportunities are created in real and authentic places where practice happens.
- **Co-construction of knowledge**. Learning happens through conversation with people in a context (i.e. ideas are interpreted within a set of cultural beliefs and influences).
- **Articulation of knowledge**. Learning is shared with others by describing new knowledge and receiving critique and an opportunity to debate.
- **Systematic reflection. Meaning, reasoning, and practice**. Once new knowledge has been constructed (shared experiences – authentic contexts), interpreted (co-construction of knowledge) and described (articulation of knowledge), it needs to be critically examined for meaning, quality of reasoning, and usefulness for practice. This is achieved through reflective strategies.

The Professional Learning through Useful Support (PLUS) Framework for Supervision

Another framework that I (Karina) developed, as an outcome of my PhD research, guides supervisors of students during fieldwork or placements. The **Professional Learning through Useful Support (PLUS) Framework** (Dancza et al., 2021) **highlights guidance that would enable supervisors to capitalise on the available educational opportunities**. Developed from practice, it offers pragmatic focal points for supervisors to make the most of their often limited time with supervisees. While designed for student learning, it could also assist supervisors more broadly. In this section we will present a modified version of the PLUS Framework in relation to professional supervision (**Figure 2.8**).

The PLUS Framework is a three-wing structure that can be positioned within the local, national, and international context of the supervisor and supervisee. The guiding principles (guide, link, and challenge) and their component actions, allow for flexibility and creativity for supervisors to come up with a range of strategies that are tailored to the supervisee and context while remaining connected with learning and teaching principles (Dancza et al., 2021). These guiding principles encase a '**supervisory time and safe space**' that reminds us of the importance of creating time for supervision and the supervisory relationship so that there is a trusting environment for open and meaningful discussion and learning.

Guide

Supervisors guide learning by supporting supervisees to **apply their existing knowledge to their current situation**. These links are needed, as applying learning from one context into another can be "rare and unpredictable" (Schell, 2018, p. 422). In addition, supervisors select specific information (e.g. how to use a coaching approach with a family member) and share it when relevant to what the supervisee is doing (e.g. when the supervisee is challenged when working with a person or they are about to enter a new therapy situation). This reflects an intentional "gradual release" of information (Evans and Guile, 2012, p. 113).

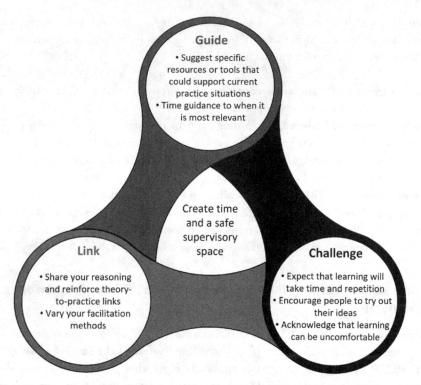

FIGURE 2.8 The Professional Learning through Useful Support (PLUS) Framework for Supervision (adapted from Dancza et al., 2021)

Link

Supervisors explicitly revisit their **own theory-to-practice links and make their decision making clear to supervisees**. For example, supervisors could engage supervisees in discussions about what they are doing, why they are doing it, how it is intended to help and when this is likely to happen. While explaining their actions and thinking, supervisors explicitly link these ideas to occupation, health, and wellbeing (i.e. occupational therapy theory). These supervision discussions reflect transformative learning theory, where supervisors engage supervisees in ongoing two-way dialogue which encourages new ideas and learning (Mezirow, 2003). Supervisors can use a variety of learning methods such as those associated with the Cognitive Apprenticeship Framework to achieve this, such as modelling, reflection, articulation, questioning, coaching, scaffolding, and fading (Collins et al., 1989; see also Figure 2.7).

Challenge

Supervisees need **time and repetition of concepts** in supervision discussions for deep learning to happen. This is particularly noticeable when novice supervisees are in new situations and need to make decisions about what to do, rather than follow established routines. Time and space are also helpful for supervisees to **try out their ideas and learn from the consequences** (provided there is adequate consideration of risk). Supervisees gain confidence when they see the results of their input and can learn from doing things for themselves.

This supportive learning space is also achieved as supervisors offer **emotional support, but also challenge supervisees to analyse, reflect, and make their own decisions** about their practice. This resonates with threshold concepts literature where learning is viewed as an embodied rather than a merely intellectual or cognitive process (Meyer and Timmermans, 2016), and it can be uncomfortable.

It is also suggested that **supervisors seek their own support** to manage the potentially emotional load associated with transformational learning. Some of the appreciative, strengths-based approaches presented earlier in this chapter may also assist supervisors to manage this positively.

Reflection is an essential skill that we need to effectively apply any of these learning and teaching frameworks and models in practice and will be the final concept we explore in this chapter.

Reflection as a learning tool

Reflection has long featured in models for learning (e.g. Schell, 2018; Kolb, 1984) and is recognised as a skill for understanding and developing capability from the complex work that we do (Yardley et al., 2012). The outcome of reflection is to create new understandings. In the case of occupational therapy supervision, we aim for positive changes in ourselves, the services we provide, and the experiences of those who access them.

Models such as Gibbs' and Rolfe's Models of Reflection provide supervisors and supervisees with ways to engage in reflective practice (Gibbs, 1998). The Gibbs model can be used after a critical incident or while debriefing about a challenging or complex scenario (see **Box 2.4**).

BOX 2.4

Components of Gibbs' Model of Refection (Gibbs, 1998)

- Description: What happened?
- Feelings: What were you thinking and feeling?
- Evaluation: What was good and bad about the experience?
- Analysis: What sense can you make of the situation?
- Conclusion: What else could you have done?
- Action plan: If the situation arose again what would you do?

Rolfe's model (Rolfe et al., 2001) uses three simple questions coined by Atkins and Murphy (1993): What? So what? and, Now what? We will return to reflection in greater detail when we discuss the skills of the supervisor in Chapter 6, but as a starting point we have some example questions that can be used across these three categories in **Box 2.5**.

BOX 2.5

Example questions from Rolfe's Model of Reflection (Rolfe et al., 2001)

- **What** happened?
- **What** were you trying to achieve?
- **What** were your feelings in that situation?
- **So what** does this tell you?
- **So what** does this indicate about your further professional development needs?
- **So what** broader issues are evident in this situation?
- **Now what** might be the consequences of this situation?
- **Now what** amendments do we need to make to your learning goals in supervision?
- **Now what** will you do next time if this situation arose again?

Reflective models are effective in structuring our thoughts and developing our reflective skills. However, to further develop our skills – including working towards and mastering critical reflexivity – the supervision environment needs to be safe for skills to develop and thrive. It is possible to achieve this even within the more traditional and hierarchical supervision structures. We invite you to read the **Reflective Story** by Madiha and Debbie **Box 2.6** where they recount their research collaboration between the United Kingdom and Pakistan. Madiha grew up in Pakistan and then moved to the United Kingdom. She worked with Debbie as the co-lead for a project supporting inclusive education (Kramer-Roy et al., 2020). Debbie was the principal investigator, and therefore the leader, responsible for coordinating and working with multiple research partners. Madiha and Debbie share their thoughts on using reflection within supervision to develop leadership skills within their different contexts.

BOX 2.6

Reflective Story by Madiha Sajid and Debbie Kramer-Roy: Developing leadership skills through reflection in supervision as part of an action research project

Madiha: In our supervision sessions, I used to share frustrations with you (Debbie), you had a very calm approach of listening to my concerns, acknowledging them (and not dismissing them), and then we'd talk about cultural differences and how we should keep this context in mind when working with the Pakistan-based team. It is ironic that I am saying this, despite being from Pakistan myself!

Debbie: As the overall project leader it was fantastic to have your consistent support. Supervision became a place for mutual feedback and sharing our reflections from a basis of trust. I think this enabled both of us to strengthen our leadership skills, both for each other and with the project team.

Madiha: I took on the leadership of a specific part of the research project which was a very enriching experience for me. Your experience, your wisdom, and your insightful approach as a supervisor were something that I found very useful. I learned one of the most important things while working with you i.e. not to rush to conclusions, but to respect cultural context, and understand how local teams work. It helped me reflect on and develop my own leadership skills and encouraged me to take on a more inclusive approach.

Debbie: I think it helped that we had worked together on a previous action research project, and we felt safe and comfortable enough to share honest reflections in supervision. For me, this was essential when leading a complex project with multiple partners in a low-income country, which came with many – expected and unexpected – challenges.

This section has presented some learning and teaching strategies that are useful in supporting professional development. In the final section of this chapter, we will consider how these general concepts that help us do supervision well need to be considered from an ethical perspective to be effective and reflective of our professional standards.

PROFESSIONAL ETHICAL CONSIDERATIONS

By their very nature, supervision and supervisory relationships are complicated. All supervisors and supervisees are responsible for understanding – and upholding – the highest ethical standards. Particularly for supervisors, this includes serving as a role model to others.

Upholding ethical standards is largely based on understanding legal, regulatory, and moral responsibilities and interpreting these dynamically into an ever-present decision-making process. This includes professional standards as well as legal and workplace standards. These are further complicated by the dual relationships between the supervisor/supervisee, the person accessing services, and the organisation (Council of State Governments, 2013). There are several ethical expectations in supervision (Substance Abuse and Mental Health Services Administration, 2009) and these are presented in **Box 2.7**.

There are many situations where ethical decision making will be required, and the answers will not be straightforward. While we cannot predict or cover all situations you may find yourself in, we will focus on some common areas within supervision:

- **Liability:** The actions or behaviours of one member of the supervisor–supervisee dyad have direct or vicarious (indirect) effects for the other.

- **Confidentiality**: Information comes to light that positions the other member of the relationship in conflict.
- **Dual relationships**: One member of the supervisor–supervisee dyad (typically the supervisor) also has another role that causes a concern or potential conflict.

BOX 2.7

Ethical expectations in supervision (adapted from Substance Abuse and Mental Health Services Administration, 2009)

- Ethics are first and foremost a way of thinking.
- Ethical issues typically arise because of conflict of some type.
- Ethical issues may have multiple answers/solutions.
- Ethical standards are a framework that typically may not tell you what to do or what not to do, requiring you to apply your judgement and decision making to complex situations.

Liability

Liability includes direct liability, such as a supervisor not trying to supervise, and vicarious liability, which is the duty of both parties to ensure care of the people accessing the services. This includes situations like a supervisor providing incorrect or inappropriate advice to the supervisee. The risk of liability increases if the supervisee has been assigned too many people on their caseload, has inadequate knowledge, or has limited access to the supervisor (Substance Abuse and Mental Health Services Administration, 2009). We introduced some ideas about safety in Chapter 1, where often people with less experience are taking on the bulk of the operational work with people who access services, and hence may be more exposed to risk. The following illustrative example **Box 2.8** highlights a situation where liability could be a concern.

BOX 2.8

Illustrative example of where liability could be a concern

You are supervising someone who has more overall experience in occupational therapy, although you have more specific experience in this area of expertise. Your unit has been considered 'underproductive' and is being closely reviewed daily. Your supervisee – who has demonstrated strong performance to this point – has been taking on a higher workload. You notice that their productivity is well beyond what is reasonable for even a seasoned practitioner in this area of specialism and that their administrative responsibilities are poorly done (documentation and communication with family, caregivers).

- What ethical concerns would you have?
- How might you go about addressing these issues?

Confidentiality

Confidentiality is a duty in the absence of a moral or ethical obligation. Whether or not there is a written contract or agreement in place between the supervisor and supervisee, confidentiality is implied for both parties to maintain relational communication, and there are limits to what is kept – and, just as importantly, what is not kept – private. Supervisors must waive confidentiality and/or intervene to prevent harm, a breach of the code of conduct or regulation or ethical standard. If information is to be shared with others, the supervisee should be informed. These standards should be maintained with all new technology. The following illustrative example **Box 2.9** highlights a situation where confidentiality could be a concern.

BOX 2.9

Illustrative example of where confidentiality could be a concern

Your supervisee is a new graduate working with people with spinal cord injury who are close in age to themselves. This is their first job, and they are very keen to help the people accessing the service. In supervision they have brought up how they feel sorry for some of the people they see as their life has been turned upside down by their accident and how they have lost friends and their vision of their future. The supervisee wants to develop rapport and has been quite successful so far. They share how some people have found them on social media and want to be connected on a personal level. Knowing that keeping connected with friends is important for recovery, the supervisee doesn't see a problem.

- What ethical concerns would you have?
- How might you go about addressing these issues?

Dual relationships

There is an inherent power differential in the supervisor–supervisee relationship. This may be additionally complicated if the supervisor also has a role (social or employment) that can compromise the professional nature of the relationship. This may be an obvious relationship (the supervisor is also the supervisee's manager in an additional capacity) or a more obscure relationship (the supervisor is the coach on the supervisee's child's sports team). Care must be taken to carefully manage this dual relationship, starting with the acknowledgement that this complication exists, and moving to an explicit agreement of how it will be managed. Our final illustrative example **Box 2.10** highlights a situation where dual relationships could be a concern.

BOX 2.10

Illustrative example of where dual relationships could be a concern

Your supervisor holds the fundraising chair position in a local chapter of a well-known and respected charitable foundation. Their latest fundraising efforts have stalled and there is a need for donations of time and money. Your supervisor has left donation and volunteer sign-up sheets in the staff office and made repeated reference to the need for help. Your supervisor is aware that you are not scheduled to work on the day of this event. Your next evaluation is due a few days after this event.

- What ethical concerns would you have?
- How might you go about addressing these issues?

Ethics in action

The best way to way to manage ethics is to uphold them. **Box 2.11** highlights best-practice tenets for supervisors and supervisees (adapted from Substance Abuse and Mental Health Services Administration, 2009). Discussing ethical concerns during your own supervision (if safe) or with trusted peers with appropriate confidentiality maintained, can also be useful to decide on the best course of action for complex situations. There may also be resources you can access, such as from professional associations or trusted organisations.

BOX 2.11

Best-practice tenets for navigating complicated situations

- Uphold the highest professional standards, including following best-practice guidelines.
- Treat all colleagues with dignity, respect, and honesty.
- Model workplace mission, vision, and philosophy.
- Demonstrate courteous and compassionate care.

CRITICAL COMMENTARY

Recipes for success in supervision … if only it was that simple!

As we write this chapter, we are aware that we have selected a few concepts that have appealed to us in some way as something that has helped us in our past supervisory experiences. We obviously cannot cover everything or go into great detail about complex topics. We hope we have given enough of an overview to spark people's interest to try out a few ideas or read more widely. We find the more we know, the more we realise we don't know. As such, we find that we apply ideas more lightly and in a considered way, rather than attempting to be an expert.

The concepts we have presented are a good starting point for thinking about what we can offer in supervision. But we rarely find all the answers in them. We don't see them as recipes for success but as a tool to progress our thinking. We still need our own careful or critical thinking to help us apply these abstract concepts into real-world situations. This is an ongoing process and, even after many years as occupational therapists, we still are learning so much.

One thing we noticed as we were writing this book was that there are not many tools aimed at the development of experienced or expert practitioners, and our understanding of the needs of people at this end of the career spectrum is limited. At this stage, people are often aware of their strengths, can harness them in their daily work, and require less detailed guidance. It made us wonder, what do people at this stage need to support their growth? Can we teach people to become expert? Or is there some as-yet not well understood mix of capabilities, mindset, opportunities (or something else) that means some people are more likely to excel? We find this makes for an interesting debate, and it may be a starting point for future research.

SUMMARY

In this chapter, we introduced some of the underpinning ideas that we will return to later in the book. We covered areas that could impact on a person's engagement in supervision when we described mindsets, motivation, and self-determination. We then proposed an appreciative, strengths-based approach to supervision and outlined specific learning and teaching principles that can be applied within supervision. Finally, we framed those concepts that help us do supervision well with an ethical lens, recognising that supervision is likely to present ethical challenges that require careful consideration.

In Chapter 3 we are excited to present our own interpretation of the critical features of supervision. The 3Cs for Effective Supervision is our attempt to consolidate the wide range of ideas that make up supervision into something that we can build on over time as we evolve our understanding of supervision.

REFERENCES

Atkins, S. and Murphy, K. (1993) 'Reflection: a review of the literature', *Journal of Advanced Nursing*, 18(8), pp. 1188–1192. doi: 10.1046/j.1365-2648.1993.18081188.x.

Bannink, F.P. (2007) 'Solution-focused brief therapy', *Journal of Contemporary Psychotherapy*, 37(2), pp. 87–94. doi:10.1007/s10879-006-9040-y.

Benner, P. (1984) *From novice to expert: excellence and power in clinical nursing practice*. Menlo Park, CA: Addison-Wesley.

Collins, A., Brown, J.S., and Newman, S.E. (1989) 'Cognitive apprenticeship: teaching the crafts of reading, writing, and mathematics', in Resnick, L.B. (ed.) *Knowing, learning, and instruction: essays in honor of Robert Glaser*. Hillsdale, NJ: Lawrence Erlbaum Associates, pp. 453–494.

Council of State Governments (2013) *Suggested state legislation: 2013 volume 72*. Available at: https://issuu.com/csg.publications/docs/2013volume (Accessed: 18 August 2021).

Craik, C. and McKay, E.A. (2003) 'Consultant therapists: recognising and developing expertise', *British Journal of Occupational Therapy*, 66(6), pp. 281–283. doi:10.1177/030802260306600608.

Dancza, K., Copley, J., and Moran, M. (2021) 'PLUS Framework: guidance for practice educators', *The Clinical Teacher*, 18(4), pp. 431–438. doi:10.1111/tct.13393.

de Shazer, S., Dolan, Y., Trepper, T., Berg, I.K., Korman, H., and McCollum, E. (2021) *More than miracles: the state of the art of solution-focused brief therapy*. 2nd edn. New York: Routledge. doi:10.4324/9781003125600.

Dreyfus, S.E. and Dreyfus, H.L. (1980) *A five-stage model of the mental activities involved in directed skill acquisition*. Berkeley, CA: California University Berkeley Operations Research Center.

Dweck, C.S. (2006) *Mindset: the new psychology of success*. New York: Random House.

Evans, K. and Guile, D. (2012) 'Putting different forms of knowledge to work in practice', in Higgs, J., Barnett, R., Billett, S., Hutchings, M., and Trede, F. (eds) *Practice-Based Education: Perspectives and Strategies*. Leiden: Brill, pp. 113–130.

Gibbs, G. (1998) *Learning by doing: a guide to teaching and learning methods*. London: Further Education Unit.

Kolb, D.A. (1984) *Experiential learning: experience as the source of learning and development*. Englewood Cliffs, NJ: Prentice-Hall.

Kramer-Roy, D., Hashim, D., Tahir, N., Khan, A., Khalid, A., Faiz, N., Minai, R., Jawaid, S., Khan, S., Rashid, R., and Frater, T. (2020) 'The developing role of occupational therapists in school-based practice: experiences from collaborative action research in Pakistan', *British Journal of Occupational Therapy*, 83(6), pp. 375–386. doi:10.1177/0308022619891841.

Leary, A. (2021) *Enhanced level practice*. PowerPoint slides, Health Education England, Birmingham.

Meyer, J.H. and Timmermans, J.A. (2016) 'Integrated threshold concept knowledge', in Land, R., Meyer, J.H.F., and Flanagan, M.T., (eds) *Threshold Concepts in Practice* (Educational Futures). Leiden: Brill, pp. 25–38.

Mezirow, J. (2003) 'Transformative learning as discourse', *Journal of Transformative Education*, 1(1), pp. 58–63. doi:10.1177/1541344603252172.

Poulsen, A., Ziviani, J., and Cuskelly, M. (2015) 'The science of goal setting', in Poulsen, A., Ziviani, J., and Cuskelly, M. (eds) *Goal setting and motivation in therapy: engaging children and parents*. London: Jessica Kingsley Publishers, pp. 28–39.

Rolfe, G., Freshwater, D., and Jasper, M. (2001) *Critical reflection for nursing and the helping professions: a user's guide*. Basingstoke: Palgrave Macmillan.

Royal College of Occupational Therapists (2021) *Professional standards for occupational therapy practice, conduct and ethics*. London: Royal College of Occupational Therapists. Available at: www.rcot.co.uk/publications/professional-standards-occupational-therapy-practice-conduct-and-ethics (Accessed: 8 May 2021).

Ryan, R.M. and Deci, E.L. (2000) 'Self determination theory and the facilitation of intrinsic motivation, social development and well-being', *American Psychologist*, 55(1), pp. 68–78.

Schell, J.W. (2018) 'Teaching for reasoning in higher education', in Schell, B.A.B. and Schell, J.W. (eds) *Clinical and professional reasoning in occupational therapy*. Philadelphia: Wolters Kluwer, pp. 417–437.

Severs, J. (2020) *Growth mindset: where did it go wrong?* Available at: www.tes.com/news/growth-mindset-where-did-it-go-wrong (Accessed: 31 May 2021).

Stavros, J.M., Torres, C., and Cooperrider, D.L. (2018) *Conversations worth having: using appreciative inquiry to fuel productive and meaningful engagement*. Oakland, CA: Berrett-Koehler Publishers.

Stoltenberg, C.D. (1998) 'A social cognitive – and developmental – model of counselor training', *The Counseling Psychologist*, 26(2), pp. 317–323. doi:10.1177/0011000098262007.

Substance Abuse and Mental Health Services Administration (2009) *Illness management and recovery: practitioner guides and handouts*. Rockville, MD: Center for Mental Health Services, Substance Abuse and Mental Health Services Administration, U.S. Department of Health and Human Services. Available at: https://store.samhsa.gov/sites/default/files/d7/priv/practitionerguidesandhandouts_0.pdf (Accessed: 14 October 2021).

Swalwell, J. and Harvey, V.S. (2017) 'Provision of supervision and school psychologists' self-care', in Thielking, M. and Tergesen, M.D. (eds) *Handbook of Australian school psychology: integrating international research, practice, and policy*. Cham: Springer, pp. 737–755. doi:10.1007/978-3-319-45166-4_39.

Yardley, S., Teunissen, P.W., and Dornan, T. (2012) 'Experiential learning: transforming theory into practice', *Medical Teacher*, 34(2), pp. 161–164. doi:10.3109/0142159X.2012.643264.

Ziviani, J. and Poulsen, A. (2015) 'Autonomy in the process of goal setting', in Poulsen, A., Ziviani, J., and Cuskelly, M. (eds) *Goal setting and motivation in therapy: engaging children and parents*. London: Jessica Kingsley Publishers, pp. 40–50.

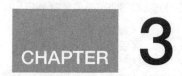

CHAPTER **3**

An introduction to the 3Cs for Effective Supervision

Karina Dancza, Stephanie Tempest, and Anita Volkert

With contributions from Joanne M. Baird, Gillian M. Taylor, Áine O'Dea, Sarah Harvey, Debbie Kramer-Roy, and Naureen Javed Hirani

CHAPTER INTENTIONS

In this chapter, we invite you to:

- Appraise the 3Cs for Effective Supervision: Connections, Content, and Continuing development
- Explore how the 3Cs for Effective Supervision can be applied within your own supervision practices
- Identify your further learning needs associated with the 3Cs for Effective Supervision.

CHAPTER HIGHLIGHTS

- Overview of the 3Cs for Effective Supervision
- Connections
- Content
- Continuing development
- Building your supervisory portfolio
- Critical commentary: Benefits and dangers of making complex things simple

CHAPTER RESOURCES

Figure

- Figure 3.1 The 3Cs for Effective Supervision

DOI: 10.4324/9781003092544-3

Boxes

- Box 3.1 Reflective Story by Gill Taylor: Applying the 3Cs for Effective Supervision
- Box 3.2 Core qualities of effective supervisory relationships
- Box 3.3 Reflective questions for developing Connections between a supervisor and supervisee
- Box 3.4 Reflective Story by Áine O'Dea: Creating Connections using a positive and encouraging environment
- Box 3.5 Questions to help supervisors and supervisees prioritise the Content of supervision
- Box 3.6 Reflective Story by Sarah Harvey: Content of effective supervision
- Box 3.7 Reflective questions for professional development
- Box 3.8 Reflective questions for your development as a supervisor and/or supervisee
- Box 3.9 Reflective Story by Debbie Kramer-Roy and Naureen Javed: Continuing development through fostering professional learning and confidence cross-culturally
- Box 3.10 Illustrative example of a new graduate occupational therapist
- Box 3.11 Illustrative example of a mid-career occupational therapist moving into a new field
- Box 3.12 Illustrative example of an experienced occupational therapist

Appendix

- Appendix 3.1 3Cs for Effective Supervision discussion tool

OVERVIEW OF THE 3CS FOR EFFECTIVE SUPERVISION

In the first two chapters, we explored definitions, common concepts, and some of the existing frameworks and models that underpin supervision. In this chapter, we would like to present our own conceptual understanding and interpretation by introducing you to the 3Cs for Effective Supervision: Connections, Content, and Continuing development (**Figure 3.1**).

The 3Cs for Effective Supervision have evolved and formed through engaging critically with the literature, reflecting on our experiences of supervision, and from the many conversations we have had together and with others – all undertaken as part of the process of writing this book. We are not introducing a new evidence-based model, rather we are presenting a framework that draws together the existing literature with our own experiences as occupational therapists, supervisors, and supervisees, and interactions with colleagues and friends. By synthesising the many and varied concepts associated with supervision into three critical features, we hope to make it more manageable for people who are embarking on supervision, often taking on this role within a time-poor context. This is a starting point for future conversations, ones we would like to continue to have with you and that we hope you will have with each other.

In this chapter, we will take each of the three components in turn and explore what makes them important throughout the supervision process. In the next three chapters we will provide detailed accounts of each of the components and offer more practical ideas for how to use them in

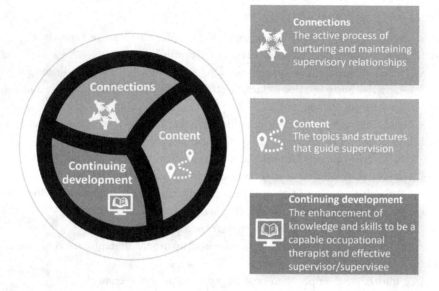

FIGURE 3.1 The 3Cs for Effective Supervision

supervision. While presented as separate components, there is overlap and interdependence. You may wish to dip in and out of these chapters depending on where in the 3Cs you see your practice strengths and areas to develop. We have also developed a summary of the tool and guidance for its use in **Appendix 3.1**.

But before we do, we would like to return to Gill who we met in Chapter 1 when we discussed the concept of creating a safe space. As part of reflecting on her supervision journey, we also asked Gill to comment on the application of the 3Cs for Effective Supervision and relate them to her own extensive experiences (**Box 3.1**).

BOX 3.1

Reflective Story by Gill Taylor: Applying the 3Cs for Effective Supervision

I am now in my sixties and, as I begin to think about retirement, I'd like to share with you my reflections on a journey through supervision which has been enlightening, inspiring, restorative, educational, strengthening, and an experience through which I learned a great deal about myself. Of equal importance is that it has provided me with a far better understanding of how supervision can be key to both personal and professional development. I hope to describe to you my reflections on this journey through supervision in relation to the 3Cs for Effective Supervision.

I now consider that I need a 'portfolio of supervision' or supervisory team, rather than relying on one person for all my supervisory needs. The flexibility and depth of the 3Cs for Effective Supervision framework means that I can apply it to any supervisory session within my portfolio. The emphasis might be on a slightly different aspect, depending on whether I am considering my professional practice or whether I just need to reflect about me (the human).

In the previous chapter, my story described my new-found 'safe space'. When I apply this to the 3Cs for Effective Supervision, I can use the framework to articulate how the safe space was created. First, **Connections** were critical through my professional relationship with myself and my supervisor. Second, **Content** was important as by applying a structure using the relevant theories and processes, we were able to create the perfect environment and safe space to explore the details of my role that worked for me and my supervisor. Finally, these **Connections** and **Content** allowed me to enhance my knowledge and skills of theories and evidence (**Continuing development**), which I could apply to my own circumstances and professional work.

Overall, as I began to have a better understanding of connections and the relational aspects of supervision and therapeutic work, I was able to utilise the relevant content and apply it to my practice in a way that advanced my expertise in being an occupational therapist.

Gill's story illustrates the 3Cs for Effective Supervision in a way that highlights the interdependent nature of each component. Another point we would like to thank Gill for sharing is the idea of a portfolio of supervision, and we will return to this concept at the end of this chapter. For now, let's look at the first C: Connections.

CONNECTIONS

The **Connection** between supervisor and supervisee refers to the relationships that impact on the supervisory process, including the relationship with your supervisor/supervisee, between supervisees (if engaging in group or peer supervision), and yourself. It is perhaps the most critical of the features as, above other factors, it has been noted as the main element influencing supervisee satisfaction (Cheon et al., 2009). Through a strong working alliance, the relationship between supervisor and supervisee(s) can mitigate other challenges experienced in the workplace.

Relationships that underpin effective supervision in occupational therapy are reported as supportive and trusting, with supervisors who are "considerate, understanding and positive" (Martin et al., 2015, p. 4), and "caring, open, collaborative, sensitive, flexible and non-judgmental"

(Rothwell et al., 2019, p. 18). These attributes are reflected in what Cassedy (2010) described as the **core qualities of the supervisory relationship**. These core qualities of empathy, congruence, acceptance, and respect are elaborated on in **Box 3.2** and are useful ways to foster the **Connections** in effective supervision.

BOX 3.2

Core qualities of effective supervisory relationships (adapted from Cassedy, 2010)

- **Empathy** – The ability to adopt another's point of view or see a situation from another's perspective. A supervisor should be able to (or attempt to) see the supervisee's perspective (and vice versa). This helps to build an understanding of their thoughts, actions, and meanings, providing additional insights into their experiences and motivations. The benefit of strong empathetic skills is that they contribute to trust and develop self-acceptance in the supervisee, which strengthens the supervisory relationship and supports learning.
- **Congruence** – This means that a supervisor is genuine and authentic, without pretence. What the supervisor thinks and feels is consistent with their actions and speech. The benefit of congruence is confidence in each other's motivations, with no sense of a hidden agenda.
- **Acceptance** – This is the ability to warmly welcome differences and positively regard others. The benefit of acceptance is the trust and safety that the supervisee experiences, which leads to freely sharing their thoughts. This allows the supervisee to be open to challenge and further exploration of issues and ideas.
- **Respect** – This requires unconditional positive regard, meaning that the supervisor is non-judgemental, and that the supervisee can enter the relationship without having to earn this positive regard. It allows the supervisor to provide honest feedback that is respectful of the supervisee and allows the supervisee to explore their thoughts and feelings without fear of rejection.

While there are many elements to supervision and qualities that make a supervisor a good match for a supervisee, these core qualities contribute to a strong, positive experience (Cassedy, 2010). As a supervisor, you may like to reflect on your personal qualities and how they align with these core qualities. As a supervisee, recognising the importance of these core qualities may help you to consider who you would like to include in your supervisory portfolio team. You can also ponder how you can support the establishment of these core qualities in your supervisory relationship. **Box 3.3** poses some questions to individually consider and perhaps discuss together as you establish a new supervisory relationship or build on an existing one.

BOX 3.3

Reflective questions for developing Connections between a supervisor and supervisee

- How can we learn to trust each other?
- What does mutual respect look like, and how do we respect differences?
- What are our own values that we bring to the supervisory relationship?
- What does 'good' feedback look like, as a supervisor and supervisee?
- What can we do when the connection is difficult to form or is challenged?

The importance of the relationship formed between supervisor and supervisee is not surprising, considering the inherent vulnerability of the supervisee, who is required to expose their uncertainties, their self-doubt, and potential gaps in their knowledge and skills. Some may argue that the supervisor is also vulnerable to judgement regarding their own knowledge and capacity to offer something useful to the supervisee, as research suggests that supervisors who are considered experts in their field are more likely to be seen as credible (Rothwell et al., 2019). The concept of vulnerability is further explored in Chapter 4.

In our next **Reflective Story** by Áine O'Dea **(Box 3.4)**, she explains how she creates Connections as a supervisor by prioritising time for supervision and designing a positive and encouraging supervisory space. As you can see, she draws on a range of supervisory strategies that we have also touched on in Chapter 2.

BOX 3.4

Reflective Story by Áine O'Dea: Creating Connections using a positive and encouraging environment

As a supervisor, I use a wide range of ways to interact with my supervisees. For example, I spend time gathering information and clarifying thoughts, and I use discussion, observation, praise, support, and prompts. Other strategies I use include explanation, monitoring, reflection, summarising, challenging, feedback, goal-setting, modelling, planning and managing the agenda, and teaching skills/ instruction (Milne et al., 2008).

I use these strategies to support the supervisee to reflect on their practice, use evidence, and align policy and service delivery. Most importantly, these strategies allow me to create a **nurturing environment** that helps to increase the supervisee's motivation to focus on what is good within their practice, and what is working well.

Using a positive and encouraging environment, I believe supervision should provide the supervisee with an opportunity to be conscious of their strengths and resources. In turn, I have found this often stimulates a conversation that facilitates new learning and increased emotional awareness, which allows the supervisee to question and explore how they might apply these resources to their next challenging situation.

From Áine's account of her supervisory style, she explains how she draws from an appreciative, strengths-based approach and focuses on what is working well for the supervisee to foster that connection between supervisor and supervisee. We agree that this is a useful approach and will return to it in Chapter 8 when we share stories about working through tensions in supervision. Connections are explored in detail in Chapter 4, but we will move on to our next C of Effective Supervision: Content.

CONTENT

The **Content** of Effective Supervision is the '**how to do it**' in practice. It refers to the structuring of the supervision sessions themselves to create an intentional process to explore the wide range of topics across managerial, educative, and supportive functions of supervision. It also includes the topics covered in supervision and will involve a range of different activities that are carefully planned, primarily to meet the needs of the supervisee, but also to fit the expectations of all partners in this relationship.

It is likely that, when you start a new supervisory relationship, you draw on the Content that you have experienced in prior supervisory relationships, such as when you were a student or an early-career therapist. Thinking that future supervision sessions will be like your previous experiences is perfectly natural. However, we would like to invite you to keep an open mind about how supervision happens and what it includes, as every situation and supervisor–supervisee relationship will be different and needs a tailored approach.

When considering the Content of supervision, there are many elements to consider such as those introduced in chapters 1 and 2. **Box 3.5** suggests a few questions to help you to think about priority Content for supervision in your own context. This could form the basis of an initial discussion during the planning of supervision or in the early sessions.

BOX 3.5

Questions to help supervisors and supervisees prioritise the Content of supervision

- What are the main purposes for supervision?
- What are some priority topics that will need to be discussed? Are managerial, educative, and supportive functions of supervision considered?
- Which supervision model(s) do we want to incorporate into the structure of supervision?
- How will we structure and document supervision sessions?
- What practical issues do we need to consider (timing, frequency, method of delivery)?
- What policies, processes, and frameworks will help inform the content of our supervision sessions (at local, regional, and national levels)?
- What level of agreement do we want between us?
- How and when will we evaluate the supervision format to check it is still working for us?

To illustrate the importance of considering a range of Content areas (structures and topics) for supervision, we have shared a **Reflective Story** by Sarah Harvey **(Box 3.6)**, as she discusses the range of Content she has benefited from in her own supervision.

BOX 3.6

Reflective Story by Sarah Harvey: Content of effective supervision

My experience of professional supervision was something to look forward to. A space to reflect, pause, take stock, and breathe. I would always have a couple of people in my caseload that I wanted to prioritise and discuss. I often chose the people that I had lost focus with, the ones that had cancelled sessions or not completed the goals they had formerly been so keen to sign up to.

Supervision allowed me to retain my occupational focus and explore the barriers that I was coming up against and consider alternative plans. My supervisor would see things that I had overlooked, question me about my approach, and get me to reflect from a different perspective to come up with my own solutions. The process gave me a confidence in my practice, assured me I was on the right track, and allowed me to develop my therapeutic communication strategies. I could learn from experiencing a safe space to have challenging conversations. I was able to use this experience to have honest conversations to ultimately benefit the people I was working with.

Sarah's story illustrates how the content of supervision was valued when, as a supervisee, she was able to choose what to discuss, and her supervisor used reflection to guide the discussions. This is one useful approach to structuring the content of supervisory sessions, and we further elaborate on these content ideas in Chapter 5. For now, we will complete our discussion of the 3Cs of Effective Supervision with a focus on the final C: Continuing development.

CONTINUING DEVELOPMENT

The third C of Effective Supervision is **Continuing development**, and refers to two aspects of professional development:

- the role of supervision in enhancing the capability of the supervisee, and
- enhancing your knowledge and skills as a supervisor and supervisee.

Within some sectors and services there is an emphasis on competence, i.e. the ability to do something at a basic threshold level. We argue that supervision can help occupational therapists go beyond just being competent. **To be capable is to practise beyond the basic threshold level**. It involves striving for excellence and developing the capability to do something well, for the benefit of those who access services, their families, and their caregivers.

Box 3.7 offers reflective questions to consider when thinking about how you might Continue your development, focusing on the first aspect – career professional development needs, i.e. relating to the supervisee's job role.

BOX 3.7

Reflective questions for professional development

- What are the supervisee's present capabilities? What is the capability of the supervisee according to the requirements of their job?
- What are the supervisee's career aspirations?
- What capabilities could be developed to enhance career development opportunities in the future?

The same rationale for professional development is true for the second aspect of Continuing development: **being a skilled supervisor and supervisee**. The better we become in these roles, the greater our potential to be effective in our occupational therapy role. With the benefits of effective supervision seen at personal, professional, and organisational levels – including as a mechanism to mitigate risk and enhance public and professional safety as discussed in Chapter 1 – we believe it is important that professional development in supervision skills is recognised as essential. **Box 3.8** highlights some areas that supervisees and supervisors may wish to consider when thinking about their knowledge and skills in their supervisory roles.

BOX 3.8

Reflective questions for your development as a supervisor and/or supervisee

- What previous knowledge, skills, and experience can I bring to the role as a supervisor or supervisee?
- How confident do I feel to support and contribute to the supervision content?
- How will I form a professional and meaningful connection with my supervisor or supervisee?
- What additional learning and development needs do I have to enhance my practice as a supervisor or supervisee?

In the following **Reflective Story** by Debbie Kramer-Roy and Naureen Javed **(Box 3.9)**, they explain how developing skills in reflection was a critical area that they worked on in supervision. The relationship was set up through a collaborative action research project, where Debbie's role was to lead and support a team of professionals in Pakistan to develop the role of occupational therapy in inclusive education. Debbie (an occupational therapist in Europe and principal investigator) explains how she supported Naureen (a teacher and participant in the research in Pakistan) and others in the setting. Debbie used reflection as a way of developing solutions collaboratively to challenges they faced, and Naureen explains how this was different from her previous experience as a supervisee, where she sought from her supervisor the 'correct answer' to the problem.

BOX 3.9

Reflective Story by Debbie Kramer-Roy and Naureen Javed: Continuing development through fostering professional learning and confidence cross-culturally

Debbie: One of the challenges of being the principal investigator of an international collaborative action research project that developed the occupational therapy role in inclusive education was managing the expectations we had of each other. Culturally, the initial expectations of the Pakistani team members were that I would be directive as the 'leader' of the project. An example of this was the online feedback I gave on the reflective logs that the team members used during their school-based activities: the logs were structured based on the action research cycle of plan–act–observe–reflect.

Reflective writing was new for most team members in the school in Pakistan, and initially they would send it back to me with the request to 'correct' the plans for interventions. I found it difficult to foster the confidence and ownership of that process in the team members, despite our in-depth conversations about the collaborative nature of our project and the value of their prior professional knowledge and skills.

It took a lot of time, with reminders that the point of me responding to their logs was to support them in **continuing their development** of reflective skills and confidence in decision making, rather than judging their professional knowledge and abilities. By only commenting on the reflective process in their log, their confidence in their own strengths and trust in their fellow team members grew. The logs were an extremely helpful tool in becoming confident action researchers, and supported the team to develop as reflective practitioners.

Naureen: Using the reflective logs helped us record all the observations, reflections, and plans we were making. The feedback we received from Debbie did not tell us if we were right or wrong in reflecting or making plans. Instead, it gave us a routine of the structure of reflection, critical thinking, and problem-solving. Hence, we were given the right to make our own decisions with the responsibility of doing the best by all means.

This was nice training hidden in the name of a collaborative action research project. It has given us the confidence to problem-solve any issue that we teachers face at school. And the best part is its continuity til the problem is resolved. All these processes gave me confidence to conduct more research and educate other teachers about conducting action research and using reflection to problem-solve.

Debbie and Naureen's story shares how their development as a supervisor and supervisee had a tangible impact on the outcomes of their collaborative action research project and wider professional work. We will explore in detail a range of ways to support development as a professional and supervisor/supervisee in Chapter 6. To conclude this chapter on the 3Cs for Effective Supervision, we return to the idea of a portfolio of supervision.

BUILDING YOUR SUPERVISORY PORTFOLIO

As a supervisee it is likely that you will need different people to work with you – depending on where you are in your career and where you wish to head. **The 3Cs for Effective Supervision can help you to select a suitable supervisory team** and be informed about where to focus your efforts to make the most of your time in supervision. It is also possible that the 3Cs can help you to see where your current supervisory arrangement is meeting your needs, and when you might consider looking for complementary supervisory experiences to address any unmet needs. This is where the idea of a supervision 'portfolio' or 'package' can be helpful, as described by Gill in her Reflective Story.

As a supervisor, the 3Cs for Effective Supervision can guide how you set up, maintain, and close your supervisory relationships. As always, the **Connection** you develop with your supervisee is a critical starting point. But, as a supervisor, you may be offering a specific focus of supervision depending on the needs and situation. For example, you may be experienced in supporting new graduate occupational therapists to transition from student to professional roles. Therefore, your supervisory relationships may be time-limited, as you guide the **Content and Continuing development** aspects of supervision to the needs of early career therapists. Keep in mind that Continuing development refers not only to the supervisee's career goals but also to both the supervisor's and supervisee's knowledge and skills in supervision.

Using the 3Cs for Effective Supervision as the basis of a supervision portfolio is probably best illustrated by examples. We will present three situations that, as editors, we are familiar with. In the first example (**Box 3.10**), we pose a potential supervisory scenario of a new graduate occupational therapist.

BOX 3.10

Illustrative example of a new graduate occupational therapist

Holly is a new graduate occupational therapist. She has an allocated professional practice supervisor who is also her line manager in the organisation. Holly uses the 3Cs for Effective Supervision to understand the expectations of the supervisory process and to have a common language with her supervisor.

The **Connection** she has with the supervisor is good, and she feels comfortable to share her successes and challenges. The **Content** is structured using a supervisory agreement, focused mainly on supportive functions and how to meet the professional competencies required for full registration. Holly is also finding areas for **Continuing development** as she realises her knowledge gaps working with the people accessing services in her setting.

Holly has expanded her portfolio of supervision to include a **peer group**. This peer group supervision is formed of other new graduates who have started in the same organisation but work across different settings. The 3Cs for Effective Supervision also help this group. Initially they prioritised making space to develop **Connections**. **Content** focuses primarily on group sharing and discussion of cases and **Continuing development** is supported through sharing relevant learning opportunities and experiences.

Our second illustrative example of the 3Cs for Effective Supervision (**Box 3.11**), is of a mid-career occupational therapist looking to move from a predominantly practice role into academia by beginning his PhD studies.

BOX 3.11

Illustrative example of a mid-career occupational therapist moving into a new field

Viktor is a mid-career occupational therapist who wants to move from a professional practice situation into an academic role. Viktor uses the 3Cs for Effective Supervision to identify his supervisory needs to help him in this transition. Viktor maintains his long-term professional practice supervisor for his existing role but adds to his supervision portfolio when he joins an academic supervisor and begins his PhD studies.

The **Content** of his academic supervision is structured using a mixture of face-to-face supervision and telesupervision. Topics are focused on the PhD process and conceptualising his research. **Continuing development** aspects of his academic supervision focus on research knowledge and skills. **Connections** with the academic supervisor support him in managing the emotional aspects of change and being introduced to a new network of people in the university.

A third element to Viktor's supervision portfolio is a peer group who are also embarking on, or are in the early stages of, their PhD studies. The 3Cs for Effective Supervision are used to structure the group discussions, prioritising Connections initially, then moving on to agreed Content reflecting the stage of their PhD and identifying further areas for Continuing development.

Our final illustrative example (**Box 3.12**), is an experienced occupational therapist who is used to being in the role of supervisor and needs to actively seek supervision from outside the organisation to meet her own supervisory needs.

BOX 3.12

Illustrative example of an experienced occupational therapist

Yu Ying is an experienced occupational therapist who is in a senior management position in a large health organisation. She has a line manager in her own organisation, but her supervision portfolio focuses on external supervision from someone in a different organisation and from a different profession. Yu Ying uses the 3Cs for Effective Supervision to explore her own **Continuing development** with the external supervisor. The **Content** of supervision offers a flexible structure that is responsive to the changing priorities and needs of her role reflecting her strategic decisions and future career progression. **Connections** remain essential for this supervisory relationship as her supervisor and peers in her own organisation offer valuable support.

When thinking back to our own careers as an editorial team, we recognised that we had never been able to gain everything we needed from a single supervisor, and that made the idea of a portfolio of supervision so helpful for us. We acknowledge that we are still working on these ideas and that they are likely to evolve as we share them with others (like you) and engage in further critical discussions. In that vein, we invite you to read our own critical commentary of our work so far, and reflect on how the 3Cs for Effective Supervision could apply to your own experiences.

CRITICAL COMMENTARY

Benefits and dangers of making complex things simple

As we embarked on writing this book, we had extensive experience of supervision in multiple settings and at multiple levels, but by no means thought of ourselves as experts. As we read others' work on supervision, from within occupational therapy but mainly from other professions (such as psychotherapy and counselling) we were fascinated by the different ideas and approaches. We reflected on our own careers and considered how, when we were in a different role as practising occupational therapists, did we have the same level of engagement with supervision literature? Honestly, our answer was: probably not!

While we do not want to assume others share our experiences, we considered how complex supervision could appear – particularly when it is part of an already busy role. This inspired us to develop the 3Cs for Effective Supervision as a potential starting point to engage in the topic of supervision. It has been necessary to ruthlessly condense ideas into a simple diagram. Our intention is not to diminish the importance of supervision or the valuable breadth and range of ideas that make supervision effective, but to make supervision more visible and accessible when it may not always be viewed as a high-status part of our role.

We have informally presented the 3Cs for Effective Supervision to our network of people within and outside of our profession, and we have refined it based on feedback received. We acknowledge that research is required to develop these initial ideas more formally. We would like to continue this conversation with anyone who is interested, as we are passionate about enhancing supervisory practices and finding new ideas to make supervision concepts accessible and implementable for all. At the core of this work is a commitment to support occupational therapists to be the best version of themselves for the safety and benefit of people who access our services.

SUMMARY

The 3Cs for Effective Supervision – Connection, Content, and Continuing development – are designed as a platform for building your own supervision portfolio. Owning your own supervision needs and seeking out opportunities to meet them both within and beyond your workplace can help you create the career you hoped you would have when you first decided to become an occupational therapist. We will build on these ideas in the next three chapters as they focus on each C in turn. While we present the concepts as three separate elements, there are many overlaps, and we feel each C provides an essential component that cannot be taken in isolation. So, with that in mind, we invite you to look through chapters 4, 5, and 6 and dive deeper into areas that you find interesting.

REFERENCES

Cassedy, P. (2010) *First steps in clinical supervision: a guide for healthcare professionals*. Maidenhead: McGraw-Hill Education.

Cheon, H.S., Blumer, M.L., Shih, A.T., Murphy, M.J., and Sato, M. (2009) 'The influence of supervisor and supervisee matching, role conflict, and supervisory relationship on supervisee satisfaction', *Contemporary Family Therapy*, 31(1), pp. 52–67. doi:10.1007/s10591-008-9078-y.

Martin, P., Kumar, S., Lizarondo, L., and VanErp, A. (2015) 'Enablers of and barriers to high quality clinical supervision among occupational therapists across Queensland in Australia: findings from a qualitative study', *BMC Health Services Research*, 15(1), pp. 1–8. doi:10.1186/s12913-015-1085-8.

Milne, D., Aylott, H., Fitzpatrick, H., and Ellis, M.V. (2008) 'How does clinical supervision work? Using a "best evidence synthesis" approach to construct a basic model of supervision', *The Clinical Supervisor*, 27(2), pp. 170–190. doi:10.1080/07325220802487915.

Rothwell, C., Kehoe, A., Farook, S., and Illing, J. (2019) *The characteristics of effective clinical and peer supervision in the workplace: a rapid evidence review*. Newcastle: Newcastle University.

Appendix 3.1: 3Cs for Effective Supervision discussion tool

The 3Cs for Effective Supervision are designed to guide supervisory practices by focusing attention on three critical elements. These prompt questions are designed to help you apply the 3Cs within supervisory discussions.

Focusing on CONNECTIONS in supervision

- How can we learn to trust each other?
- What does mutual respect look like, including how do we respect differences?
- What are our own values that we bring to the supervisory relationship?
- What does 'good' feedback look like, as a supervisor and supervisee?
- What can we do when the connection is difficult to form or is challenged?

Notes:

Focusing on CONTENT of supervision

- What are the main purposes for supervision?
- What are some priority topics that will need to be discussed? Are managerial, educative, and supportive functions of supervision considered?
- Which supervision model(s) do we want to incorporate into the structure of supervision?
- How will we structure and document supervision sessions?
- What practical issues do we need to consider (timing, frequency, method of delivery)?
- What policies, processes and frameworks will help inform the content of our supervision sessions (at local, regional, and national levels)?
- What level of agreement do we want between us?
- How and when will we evaluate the supervision format to check it is still working for us?

Notes:

(Continued)

Focusing on CONTINUTING DEVELOPMENT in supervision

- What are the supervisee's present capabilities? What is the capability of the supervisee according to the requirements of their job?
- What are the supervisee's career aspirations?
- What capabilities could be developed to enhance career development opportunities in the future?
- What previous knowledge, skills, and experience can I bring to the role as a supervisor or supervisee?
- How confident do I feel to support and contribute to the supervision content?
- How will I form a professional and meaningful connection with my supervisor or supervisee?
- What additional learning and development needs do I have to enhance my practice as a supervisor or supervisee?

Notes:

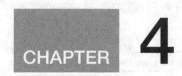

CHAPTER 4

Making and maintaining connections within the supervisory relationship

Stephanie Tempest, Vicki Craig, and Anita Volkert

With contributions from Charmaine Green, Carol-Ann Howson, Monica Moran, and Lenny Papertalk

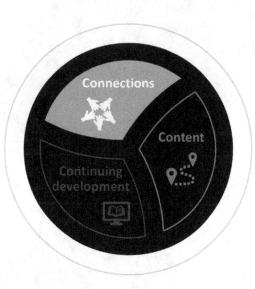

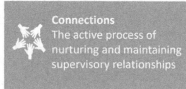

Connections
The active process of nurturing and maintaining supervisory relationships

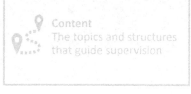

Content
The topics and structures that guide supervision

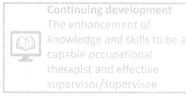

Continuing development
The enhancement of knowledge and skills to be a capable occupational therapist and effective supervisor/supervisee

DOI: 10.4324/9781003092544-4

CHAPTER INTENTIONS

In this chapter, we invite you to:

- Consider supervision from a relational perspective
- Evaluate the importance of self-care within the supervisory relationship
- Explore some of the concepts involved in understanding yourself as a supervisor or supervisee within the supervisory relationship
- Review the concept of self-care from an organisational perspective
- Examine the concept of inclusive supervision.

CHAPTER HIGHLIGHTS

- Self-care as a relational concept
- Concepts to aid connection with yourself within the supervisory relationship, including understanding defence mechanisms, unhelpful or destructive roles in supervision, and permeability as a practitioner
- Inclusive supervision to maintain connections
- Critical commentary: Finding it difficult to look after ourselves in the helping and caring professions

CHAPTER RESOURCES

Figures

- Figure 4.1 Professional and personal energy analogy
- Figure 4.2 Malan's Triangle of Conflict
- Figure 4.3 The Drama Triangle
- Figure 4.4 Behaviours and characteristics of the permeable supervisor/supervisee
- Figure 4.5 Differences between cultural humility and cultural competence

Boxes

- Box 4.1 Exploring what self-care means to you
- Box 4.2 Editor's Reflective Story: Writing about self-care for an audience of occupational therapists
- Box 4.3 Reflective Story by Carol-Ann Howson: Elegant challenge as a self-care activity
- Box 4.4 Identifying your own defence mechanisms
- Box 4.5 Identifying examples of the roles you play in supervision
- Box 4.6 Editor's Reflective Story: Being a permeable supervisee (even before I knew what that was)

SELF-CARE AS A RELATIONAL CONCEPT

In this chapter we will be focusing on the first C for Effective Supervision, **Connections**. We consider the idea that self-care is a relational concept involving connections with yourself and with your supervisor/supervisee. As an important starting point to connecting with others, we will explore what we mean by connecting with and understanding ourselves, and why this is relevant to you as a supervisee and supervisor. We will explain how, to support other people effectively, we need to understand and take care of ourselves, as an ethical requirement. We will outline ways this can be done and highlight the central role that effective supervision plays in keeping us safe and secure. This is essential. When professionals feel secure in practice, we (the public) can be confident in the services we access (Harding, 2021).

As an occupational therapist, you act as a container for others, to support people, their families, and carers who access the services you provide. You will also act as a container for colleagues through formal supervision or line management responsibilities, or as part of an informal professional network. This requires a significant amount of professional and personal energy.

It may be helpful to think of yourself in the same way as you think of your mobile phone (see **Figure 4.1**). If the battery is full, it functions well. You may still need to use it towards the end of the day when the power is diminishing, but there is a facility to turn on the low-battery function to enable you to perform the basic tasks. You know that to preserve the battery of your phone, you need to make sure you do not have too many applications open at the same time. And you will put it into sleep mode to recharge it because you know it will function better the next day if you do. Similarly, you also need time to recharge and know where the best charging points are, to be a container for yourself so you can provide safe and effective services.

So, let's start this chapter with **Box 4.1** and a series of questions on the topic of self-care, for which there are no right or wrong answers.

We are asking these questions to start with because we are aware that, in this chapter, we might be asking a lot from you as a reader and learner. You may find that you are revisiting your understanding of self-care and some of this may feel uncomfortable, as we seek to challenge you to think about yourself as 'your own first client' – a phrase used within the counselling profession to help new counsellors understand and acknowledge the importance of self-care.

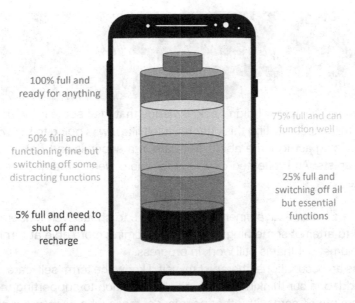

100% full and
ready for anything

75% full and can
function well

50% full and
functioning fine but
switching off some
distracting functions

25% full and
switching off all
but essential
functions

5% full and need to
shut off and
recharge

FIGURE 4.1 Professional and personal energy analogy

BOX 4.1

Exploring what self-care means to you

- When you think of the phrase 'self-care', what are the first five things that spring to mind?
- From your list of five things, how many relate to you and how many relate to the self-care of others? What else do you see in your list?
- Say the phrase 'self-care' out loud. What feelings are evoked that you are able to notice? There may be a mix, e.g. a feeling of comfort but with a level of cynicism? Or a feeling of familiarity with the term but an awareness that you are detached from thinking about applying the concept to yourself? You may feel validated that we are talking about the legitimacy of taking care of yourself, because it's something you have always been passionate about, but feel others may not take it as seriously as you.

This chapter does not provide a checklist or a recipe for success on how to maintain a supervisory relationship or how to look after yourself. Rather, it will present a set of ideas and concepts, and we invite you to reflect on these by yourself and within supervision. Central to our discussion is the need to view **self-care as a relational concept** and one that is based on trust: trust in yourself, derived from knowing yourself, and trust built through working together in the supervisory relationship. With this in mind, we invite you to read the **Editor's Reflective Story** and Steph's account of starting out on the task of writing this chapter (**Box 4.2**).

BOX 4.2

Editor's Reflective Story: Writing about self-care for an audience of occupational therapists

I (Steph) would be lying if I didn't acknowledge that I felt some nervousness as I started to think about writing this chapter. It felt like it was going to be a challenge and a balancing act to write about self-care in a supervision book for occupational therapists. As I reflected on this, I felt there were three main reasons for my unease.

First, I have a rather active inner critic, who likes to shout even louder when I'm about to attempt something new. I am becoming more able at turning down the volume, but that is still work in progress.

Second, as an occupational therapist myself, I know the term 'self-care' is deeply embedded in our thinking, albeit mainly in relation to supporting the 'doing' aspects of self-care with other people, i.e. those who access our services. I felt concerned that you, as a reader, might think I was going to try to tell you things you already knew. This could be misconstrued as patronising on my part. However, in this chapter we are going to be talking about self-care in a very different way, a relational way, and for that I felt excited.

The third reason for my nervousness is the fact that we are writing this book at a point in time when a global pandemic remains very real and present in our world. I find myself with a growing sense of discomfort at the predominant self-care discourse in the mainstream media and the social consciousness (in the United Kingdom but perhaps elsewhere too), which focuses on self-care primarily at the level of the individual – often linked to pushing the need for personal resilience, positive thinking, and a change in mindset. I do not want to amplify further the individuality of self-care in this chapter and be a part of a dominant narrative that I perceive to be unhelpful.

However, a discussion on the need to build inclusive structures and systems where everyone can thrive is beyond the scope of this chapter. With that in mind, I invite you to read this chapter alongside Chapter 9, which focuses on the governance and strategic requirements to develop supervision practices, in part to aid self-care of the workforce.

So, what have I done to manage my nervousness? I have built a writing team; it is a form of relational self-care support for myself. I chose to connect with others from within and beyond our profession – specifically people who I hold in high respect and, most importantly, people I trust.

Vicki Craig is a counsellor and psychotherapist, part of a profession which views supervision as a way of life and encourages both supervisor and supervisee to invest time in building and maintaining the connections in this key relationship. Vicki is also my sister. We have experiences over four decades in navigating relational and restorative aspects of self-care, which includes continuing to learn from the mistakes we make along the way.

Anita Volkert is a new connection, a collaborator, and occupational therapy colleague. We were brought together to work on this book by Karina, for which I am eternally grateful. Anita is very skilled at providing gentle sense-checking and honest perspectives which are delivered with care.

Carol-Ann Howson is a social worker and academic with whom I first connected as a fellow PhD student and as an academic colleague. I continue to experience first-hand the restorative capacity of her wisdom and knowledge.

I have connected with the final team members purely through their writing contributions – Monica Moran, Lenny Papertalk, and Charmaine Green. We have never met, but their words and stories have also helped to manage my nervousness at writing this chapter, to the point that I'm now looking forward to you reading it.

CONCEPTS TO AID CONNECTION WITH YOURSELF WITHIN THE SUPERVISORY RELATIONSHIP

Continuing to explore the Connections component of our 3Cs for Effective Supervision, in this section we will be considering some of the ways to know yourself through the concepts of elegant challenge, defensive mechanisms, the roles we play in supervision (some of which are unhelpful), and the concepts of vulnerability and permeability.

Becoming an effective supervisor or supervisee through connecting with, and taking care of, yourself

As a counsellor (Vicki), my professional philosophy is underpinned by my personal belief that we exist in the context of relationships. That is, the relationship we have with ourselves as well as with other people. The nature of my work necessitates that I know myself well enough to reduce the risk that my own values and assumptions do not negatively affect my work with people or, as we like to say, my own baggage does not thrust itself into another person's world.

I was required to complete personal counselling therapy as part of my training, and I saw this as self-care. Alongside that, I had a supervisor with whom I continue to work since qualifying as a counsellor. My supervisor sits outside of the organisations in which I work to provide ongoing support for every aspect of my portfolio career. Of primary importance is that the relationship I have with my supervisor also supports me to keep in touch with myself. However, there is an important boundary between therapy and supervision; **supervisors are not required**

to be therapists to their supervisees. Rather, the role should provide a restorative function that may include considering or signposting for counselling and other forms of support elsewhere as an option.

Shohet and Shohet (2020) include 'knowing yourself' as a core proposition and principle of supervision, one which is relevant to anyone, whatever their work or profession. Let us look at how we may begin to do this through a fictional, but recognisable, person called Mary in the **Reflective Story** by Carol-Ann **(Box 4.3)**.

BOX 4.3

Reflective Story by Carol-Ann Howson: Elegant challenge as a self-care activity

Mary was a newly qualified social worker, and she was struggling to know what to do to support Jonas, a person recently allocated into her caseload, who presented with multiple and complex needs. Despite Mary recognising that she needed help, she wanted to cancel her upcoming supervision meeting or pretend she had double-booked herself. She felt anxious that she would be asked about the work she was doing with Jonas and that she would be left feeling exposed because she didn't know where to start. However, Mary's supervisor (who was also her line manager) spoke to her the day before supervision and reminded her about their meeting, so she felt she had to attend.

Mary considered why she wished to avoid supervision when she needed help. She reflected on her experience of supervision to date, and felt she derived no benefits from her meetings as she was talked down to and endured sarcastic remarks about the issues and concerns she raised. For example, she said to her supervisor that on one of her visits she was scared of the dog at the house, which barked aggressively while approaching her. While laughing, her supervisor's response was "You should have just barked louder, and it would have stopped."

Mary explored her supervisor's reaction and comment with a friend from another team who knew the supervisor. This friend, also a social worker, told Mary about the concept of **elegant challenge, a technique which involves (1) being clear and focused in your description of an event, (2) identifying what you want to achieve as an outcome from raising it, and (3) expressing it in a way that allows for it to be well received**. Mary's friend encouraged her to think about how the concept could be used to address the situation. However, Mary felt scared, as she had just joined the team and her colleagues were always singing the praises of the manager, whom they described as relaxed and humorous.

While waiting for her supervisor to arrive for their meeting, Mary became so anxious that she had to rush to the bathroom to be physically sick. Several thoughts crossed Mary's mind. First, she thought of telling her supervisor that she was leaving the job. Second, she thought of cancelling the meeting because she was feeling unwell. Finally, she thought about the concept of elegant challenge. So, when the time came for supervision, Mary decided to challenge her supervisor elegantly.

Mary composed herself and started by saying that she enjoyed working in the team, but she was anxious about supervision. At that point, her supervisor asked what was making her anxious. Reflecting on her experiences of previous supervision meetings, using a conciliatory tone, Mary carefully outlined all her concerns and spoke about how they had adversely impacted her confidence to practise. She ended by expressing a hope that they could work together to find a way of making supervision a more positive experience.

Mary's supervisor listened until she had finished and paused to consider what had been said and heard. A discussion ensued in an atmosphere of mutual respect and effective communication. The supervisor demonstrated a genuine concern about Mary's thoughts by responding sensitively and offering an immediate apology, which Mary accepted. Both agreed to move forward, recognising their respective roles within the supervision process. The supervisor acknowledged Mary's constructive approach and commended her on the way she had raised her concerns.

Before we look at the supervisory relationship, let's consider Mary's responses to the situation. Mary is feeling deflated, anxious, scared, and in response to these uncomfortable feelings, she has an urge to avoid the meeting with her supervisor to the point where she is physically sick at the thought of attending. The desire to avoid difficult situations, people, or relationships is certainly something I recognise, and we can consider this response through the psychological concept of defence mechanisms.

Understanding defence mechanisms

The world of psychotherapy loves a triangle, and Malan's Triangle of Conflict (1995 [1979]; **Figure 4.2**) can help us to understand the process of what is happening for Mary in our example. The premise, as represented by the diagram, is that when we experience difficult feelings or impulses, we feel anxious, and to reduce the anxiety, we employ a defence mechanism to protect ourselves from feeling this way. Although this sounds straightforward, because we may have been using these strategies from an early age, we may not even notice when this process is fired, hence the term 'unconscious'. When we act unconsciously, this happens either on the edge or outside of our awareness. So, the first step in knowing ourselves is to understand the personal defences that we use to reduce feelings of anxiety.

Before we return to Mary, it is worth noting that defences are a normal and often necessary part of life. Defences can be referred to as a 'psychic skin' (Lemma, 2016) that allows us to cope

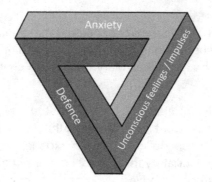

FIGURE 4.2 Malan's Triangle of Conflict (adapted from Malan, 1995 [1979])

with the inevitable pitfalls in life. They can also be healthy, if used appropriately, for example the role of humour or deliberately switching off to engage in healthy occupations to manage your own wellbeing. They can also help us to maintain our professionalism in the moment, for example, the ability to compartmentalise a difficult work situation until you can talk to a trusted friend or colleague. However, if we are not aware of the extent or how often we are compartmentalising difficult situations, then our emotional wellbeing can be negatively affected. Defences become an issue when we apply them too rigidly and too often without recognising them or their consequences.

Fortunately, Mary understands herself well enough, and speaks with a friend before returning to supervision. But let us consider some other possible outcomes, illustrated by other common defence mechanisms:

- Mary could have continued to **rationalise** that she could miss supervision because she wasn't gaining any benefit. Rationalising is a defence mechanism that involves making something acceptable to ourselves when actually it isn't.
- Mary could **displace** her thoughts and feelings about her supervisor towards another person. Displacement is a defence mechanism which results in us taking our frustrations out on someone close to us because it feels safer than confronting the real person or issue.
- Mary's physical sickness can also be considered a possible defence response. **Conversion** is a defence mechanism that can see emotional responses presenting physically.

These are just a few examples of the more recognisable defence mechanisms. I would also include **intellectualisation** within this group. In writing this chapter, I spent too many hours searching for academic sources, which I realise now was wasted time. I may have been better off accepting the anxiety and just getting on with the writing. In intellectualising, we place too much emphasis on thinking when we experience difficult feelings. Of importance is to recognise our emotional responses so we give ourselves more choice over how to respond. This supports us to take care of ourselves and develop more healthy coping mechanisms at times of stress. I see supervision as one of my healthy coping mechanisms but invite you to think about your own by considering the questions in **Box 4.4**.

> **BOX 4.4**
>
> ## Identifying your own defence mechanisms
>
> - How familiar is the concept of defence mechanisms for you?
> - Can you identify some of your own emotional responses in the defence mechanisms listed?
> - What other defence mechanisms do you use?
> - Which of your defence mechanisms are helpful and which ones might you need to recognise in greater depth?
> - How comfortable do you feel about sharing your defence mechanisms within supervision as a supervisor or supervisee?

You may now be at the stage of reading this chapter where it all feels good in theory but vastly different from the practical reality of your own supervisory experiences. Or you may be feeling over- or underwhelmed by the emphasis we are placing on you and your ability to know yourself and to take care of yourself at work. Or we may have got it just right. Whatever you are feeling right now, we invite you to take a moment to capture, define, and own the emotions and thoughts. And know that we are grateful that you have held your curiosity to the place that you are still with us, in reading and thinking about the things we are sharing with you.

With this in mind, we appreciate that there are many other concepts and models to support you in developing deeper connections with yourself, to enhance your relational self-care skills. We aim to find a balance in this chapter where we do not present an entire textbook on these concepts, nor do we want to present them in a superficial manner that would not do them justice. Therefore, we would like to discuss three more concepts – unhelpful or destructive roles, vulnerability, and permeability – and invite you to consider them as concepts to inform self-care activities when looking after yourself as a supervisee and/or supervisor.

Unhelpful or destructive roles in supervision

We all play different roles within our personal and professional relationships. There are many roles that are helpful, e.g. coach, facilitator, supporter. There are many that are not, and we sometimes act out these roles without consciously knowing we are doing so. Before we continue this section, it is important to emphasise that we are not talking about you as an individual or making comments on your personality traits. To put this in context, think about your favourite actor and all the characters you have seen them play throughout their career. Think about the complexity within each character and appreciate that your favourite actor is playing several roles. That is what we are referring to in this section – the roles we either consciously or unconsciously play within supervision, with particular focus on three unhelpful ones.

In 1968, Stephen Karpman published his theory of the Drama Triangle. The basic premise is that there are three potentially destructive roles that can be enacted within relationships (see

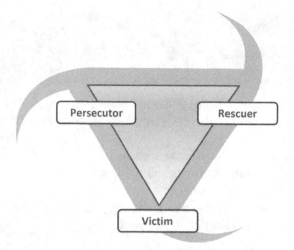

FIGURE 4.3 The Drama Triangle (adapted from Karpman, 1968)

Figure 4.3) and in this case we are applying the theory to supervisory relationships. The victim is deliberately at the inverted base of the triangle – a role which involves feeling helpless, hopeless, and powerless. In contrast, the persecutor is controlling, blaming, and superior. The rescuer role, which on the face of it may look helpful, is just as destructive. The rescuer role involves constantly 'helping out', often when it is not needed and when others could do things for themselves. Therefore, it creates an unnecessary dependency, reinforcing the victim as weak and preventing them from experiencing, learning from, and being empowered by making their own choices.

Left unchecked and sometimes unconsciously, we can all inhabit all the roles within Karpman's Drama Triangle, and sometimes even within the course of one interaction. Imagine if Mary had allowed herself to feel powerless (victim), convincing herself that her supervisor was always going to be sarcastic, that there was nothing she could do about it (because it wasn't the first time someone had spoken to her like that) and then decided to leave her job. Mary's supervisor could have continued to play the role of persecutor, by not listening to Mary's concerns, dismissing her feelings, and implying that Mary herself was the problem. Or perhaps Mary's friend, to feel needed themselves, had intervened by talking to Mary's supervisor (rescuer) but, then complained to colleagues in the office about how much support they felt they needed to give Mary at the expense of getting on with their own work (persecutor/victim).

Consider the questions in **Box 4.5** in relation to yourself, and then think about them in the context of your supervision and the organisation in which you work (if applicable).

BOX 4.5

Identifying examples of the roles you play in supervision

- How familiar are the three roles in the Drama Triangle?
- Can you identify some of your own moments where you have acted the roles, including during supervision?

- What other roles do you play?
- Which of your other roles are more helpful, and how could they help you over-come some of the more unhelpful roles you play?
- How could you use the concepts in the Drama Triangle within your profes-sional interactions and relationships? Do you feel you could share and discuss it within supervision as a supervisor or supervisee?

While we have focused on the Drama Triangle in relation to individuals and within the supervisory relationship, it is important to acknowledge that the roles can also be enacted at an organisational level, e.g. working in a blame culture is linked to the persecutor role. Another example of the persecutor role at an organisational level is one that we are anecdotally hearing more about – the growing pressure for greater individual resilience in response to constant change and workplace pressure. This places the responsibility solely with the person, without acknowl-edging the role of organisational policies and structures in developing a conducive and responsive working environment.

For a detailed discussion of a solution-focused approach to living outside of the Drama Trian-gle, we invite you to search for 'Drama Triangle', preferably within the parameters of an academic literature search. This will take you on a journey exploring many other triangle-based theories, e.g. Winner's Triangle (Choy, 1990) focusing on empowerment and relationship dynamics.

Vulnerability

We have already met vulnerability in this chapter. To return to Mary, she displayed courage in showing her vulnerability with her supervisor when she spoke about how she felt and the help she needed. Fortunately, her supervisor responded non-defensively, and they were able to move forward positively.

When you look at dictionary definitions for vulnerability, they suggest this is a concept that we should run away from. Vulnerability is defined as a weakness or an area where you are exposed or at risk – a noun that describes a susceptibility to attack or harm. And yet here it is, featured in a chapter on taking care of yourself and maintaining Connections within the super-visory relationship.

The work of Brene Brown, among others, challenges us to think about the definition of vul-nerability differently. As a social worker and academic, Brown has spent over 25 years researching the interrelated concepts of vulnerability, shame, courage, and empathy. Her online talk on 'The power of vulnerability' (Brown, 2010) has been viewed nearly 55 million times and, rather than repeat the key points here, readers are encouraged to take 20 minutes out of their day to listen to it wholeheartedly.

Brown concludes and encourages us to work with the discomfort that vulnerability and shame give us, so we have capacity for courage and empathy. We are invited to choose courage over comfort. This also helps us to be realistic about ourselves and own our imperfections – things we all have, yet sometimes seek to hide. Central to this is **believing in the concept of 'good enough'** which Brown argues is an act of self-care in itself. So, by embracing vulnerability, by acknowledging and attending to shame, and aiming for good enough, we are kinder and gentler to ourselves and the people around us – including those we serve. This places the discussion firmly within professional, ethical, and safe practice.

Before we move on, we want to acknowledge that much of the literature and our own background experience has been within the British or Australian cultures, where questioning, critique, and openness for discussion with people – including with people who are more experienced within the workplace – are largely accepted or tolerated. We appreciate and acknowledge that there are situations and cultures beyond ours that have different norms and values which will influence how people conduct themselves and react to discomfort, challenge, and vulnerability.

While we can all find much in common, differences in contexts and personal connections are also inevitable, and it is essential to recognise these, particularly in the supervisory relationship. Later in the chapter, Monica, Lenny, and Charmaine will share their journey in understanding different norms and values within their supervisory relationships, and what they have done so far to navigate them successfully. Whatever your situation and context, it is worth reflecting on your own level of comfort or discomfort in asking for help and support, that of your supervisor/supervisee and the system in which you work.

Permeability as a practitioner

As with all relationships, the supervisory relationship is co-created, and it is worth taking the time to get to know yourself and each other within it. We saw the beginnings of this happening with Mary, as she started to become more open with her supervisor as part of her elegant challenge. Hopefully, the relationship building between Mary and her supervisor continues; Mary could share her defence mechanisms so her supervisor can support her restoratively when these emerge again in her work. Equally, Mary's supervisor could be open to developing greater self-awareness and a willingness to change themselves, to develop a safer supervisory space for Mary. This is in the context of remembering that when practitioners feel secure, people who access their services can have greater confidence in them.

Permeability, or more specifically, the concept of the 'permeable practitioner', grew from research exploring health and care professionals' experiences of supervision (Harding, 2019). Permeable practitioners expect and anticipate uncertainty within their practice. They also actively seek to learn from uncertainty, manage it, or resolve it (Harding, 2019), which also involves adopting the growth mindset we described in Chapter 2. The concept has since featured in multiprofessional guidance for workplace supervision, including for advanced practitioners (Health Education England, 2020).

In the context of this chapter, we would like to focus on the idea of developing ourselves as **permeable supervisors or supervisees**, rather than explore the broader requirements in relation to the work we do with the people who access our services. Within supervision, we should expect and anticipate uncertainty, seek to learn from it, and apply that learning to strengthen the connections we have with others. Importantly, and as part of effective supervision practice, we need to feel we are agents of change who can influence what happens to us through our actions.

Seven behaviours and characteristics are evident in permeable practitioners (as described in **Figure 4.4** in relation to supervision, adapted from Harding, 2019). The characteristics are

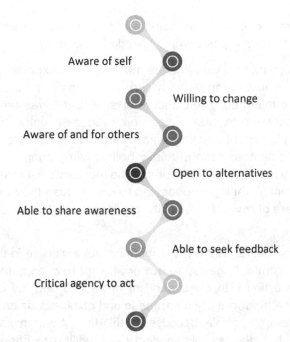

Aware of self

Willing to change

Aware of and for others

Open to alternatives

Able to share awareness

Able to seek feedback

Critical agency to act

FIGURE 4.4 Behaviours and characteristics of the permeable supervisor/supervisee (adapted from Harding, 2019)

interrelated and need to be developed alongside each other. Through the research (with occupational therapists, physiotherapists, and speech and language therapists), Harding concludes there is a spectrum of permeability for everyone, and how sometimes we act with more or less permeability. Too much permeability can foster dependency; and being impermeable leaves us struggling to cope with change. Effective supervision can act as a safe space for us to explore our permeable characteristics. Equally, exploring the characteristics together within supervision (as outlined in Figure 4.4) may help to develop effective Connections.

As an example of how the behaviours and characteristics of the permeable supervisor/supervisee can help us understand our reactions to situations, we invite you to read the next **Editor's Reflective Story (Box 4.6)**. Think about this story in relation to Mary's, as part of identifying the characteristics that are needed to challenge elegantly.

BOX 4.6

Editor's Reflective Story: Being a permeable supervisee (even before I knew what that was)

I (Steph) can now reflect on my varying levels of permeability throughout my career. An early example is from my experiences on a practice placement as a 19-year-old student occupational therapist. I was particularly hesitant to be a 'permeable practitioner' in supervision as I was also being assessed by my supervisor. I felt this was a place where I needed to 'perform'.

During the placement, I noticed in team meetings how experienced and qualified colleagues would compete with and undermine each other, and these behaviours were tolerated. I felt uncomfortable, but I was reluctant to say anything in supervision in case I was perceived as causing trouble. A few weeks into the placement, the dynamics started to be directed towards me as a student. I remember sitting, quietly boiling with anger, embarrassment, and shame in a team meeting, after one of the therapists said they were going to give the student all their photocopying to do because they were much too busy. I was **aware of myself**, yet I still did not feel able to say anything to my supervisor.

The comments persisted, as did my discomfort. As a student in the team, I did not feel I had the **critical agency to act** or attempt to change the behaviours. But, as the connection with my supervisor developed and my courage grew, I challenged myself to **share my awareness** and observations and seek advice from my supervisor (especially because by this time it was my final week, so it felt safer too). Nonetheless this showed I was **willing to change and seek feedback**.

If I'm honest, the discussion in supervision could have gone better (if I'd met Carol-Ann earlier in my career and knew more about elegant challenge it would have helped!). I was defensive and I let some of my anger show in an unhelpful way, which made it harder for my supervisor to receive. However, they explained the situation from the staff member's perspective – the pressure they were under, the staff shortages, and their recently rejected promotion application. I was **open to alternatives** to explain their behaviour. I learned a valuable lesson about the need to be **aware of and for others** in part to understand team dynamics. My supervisor coached me in how I should approach the staff member (notice that they did not seek to 'rescue' by doing it for me). Feeling empowered, yet still very nervous, I chose a quiet time to have a conversation with the team member which went well. I was grateful for the way they handled the conversation, and I was able to finish the placement feeling positive about the experience.

I remember the interaction clearly, 27 years later, as seen by the reality that I wanted to share it with you. It proved to be a pivotal learning point in my career. And now I can revisit it and reflect on it using the characteristics of the permeable practitioner and the concept of elegant challenge. Using the theory and evidence, I now have a deeper understanding of the multiple factors that contributed to my discomfort on that placement many years ago.

Before we move on to our next section, we would like to invite you to think of a situation that has been memorable in your career and consider how permeable you were within it, using the questions in **Box 4.7**.

BOX 4.7

How permeable are you?

- Think about each characteristic of a permeable practitioner. Which ones do you feel are your strengths and which would you like to develop further?
- Identify situations where your levels of permeability have varied and think about what might have contributed to that.
- How could you use the concept of the permeable practitioner within your supervision sessions either as a supervisor or supervisee?
- Consider one or two small actions you can take in the next week or month to develop yourself as a permeable practitioner.

This section has focused on you as a supervisor or supervisee and has explored concepts to support you to **make effective Connections with yourself**. As we close this section, it feels like a good opportunity to reiterate that occupational therapy supervision does not involve doing the actual self-work related to taking care of yourself, as we have discussed. **We are not trained counsellors, and our boundaries lie in recognising, supporting, and signposting if required**. We encourage any occupational therapist supervisee or supervisor who recognises any disconnect or rupture in how they look after themselves to seek professional support and guidance. We know there are many of us who do just that and find it a powerful, developmental, and affirming experience.

INCLUSIVE SUPERVISION TO MAINTAIN CONNECTIONS

Inclusive supervision is based on four tenets: **creating safe spaces, cultivating holistic development, demonstrating vulnerability, and building capacity in others** (Wilson et al., 2019). Underpinning the work towards inclusivity is the need to focus on the relationships and, as we have discussed, this includes the relationship we have with ourselves as well as the relationship with our supervisor/supervisee.

The **responsibility to improve supervisory practices does not lie purely with us as individual practitioners**. Strategic emphasis and organisational policies are essential to drive through meaningful change. For example, Brown et al. (2020) argue that inclusive supervision requires an **identity-conscious approach** and propose nine core strategies including managing power, acting with courage, and engaging with conflict. Of importance is the emphasis on doing this work across the system, including with the individual, within the supervisory process, and at an organisational level. We will return to the nine strategies for an identity-conscious approach in Chapter 9, as part of discussing how policy can drive the work towards creating conditions for effective supervision.

In this section, we will continue our focus on the individual and the supervisory relationships. We are now going to focus our attention on what it means to **keep and maintain Connections as supervision progresses**. And we have chosen to do this by sharing a detailed story of cross-cultural supervision with an Irish Australian woman (**Monica**) and two Australian Aboriginal women (**Lenny and Charmaine**). Together they identify the factors that maintain connections within their specific supervisory relationship. We invite you to find somewhere comfortable to sit or create your own conditions where you know you will be able to read and listen wholeheartedly. We suggest you read the story through at least twice. On the first occasion, read it with the purpose of understanding the content from Monica, Lenny, and Charmaine's perspectives. On subsequent occasions, allow your mind to make connections with your own experiences and context.

BOX 4.8A

Reflective Story by Monica Moran, Lenny Papertalk, and Charmaine Green: Inclusive, cross-cultural supervision.

Part 1: Background

This reflective story was developed by Monica, an Irish Australian woman, and Lenny and Charmaine, two Australian Aboriginal women. All three of us live in rural Western Australia and work for the same organisation. Our ideas, recommendations, and reflections are based on our experiences of working together in particular geographic and cultural contexts, and on our life experiences of living and working in Australia. Monica has lived in Australia since 1986. Lenny and Charmaine have lived in Australia for their entire lives. We present our experiences and recommendations to you as a starting point for your thinking, sharing of thoughts, and discussions on supervision practice with and for Aboriginal people wherever they may reside.

Across the world, Indigenous peoples have experienced a long tail of disadvantage stemming from colonisation and subjugation endeavours that were enacted over hundreds of years, and in some regions of the world are still being enacted.

Colonising societies almost universally imposed sociopolitical controls on First Nations communities that result in loss of culture and language, dislocation from and theft of lands, educational and vocational disadvantage, removal of artefacts, theft of wages, and minimisation of the bodies of knowledge valued by Indigenous people.

Aboriginal and Torres Straits Islander people, also known as Australian First Nations people, are acknowledged as the oldest known civilisation on Earth with evidence of continuous occupation dating back over 60,000 years. A little over 230 years ago, Australia was colonised as a penal colony and then as land for

expansion by European settlers. The sovereign rights of the continuous inhab-
itants were ignored, and Aboriginal and Torres Straits Islander people were not
recognised as citizens of Australia until the national referendum of 1967.

That resulted in the recognition of Aboriginal and Torres Straits Islander people as
citizens, and there have been gradual improvements in educational, vocational,
and social circumstances, although many inequities still exist. For example, the
gap in life expectancy between Aboriginal and Torres Straits Islander people and
the rest of the Australian population remains around ten years – despite ongoing
efforts to close this gap. A more promising outcome is the increase in Aboriginal
and Torres Straits Islander students finishing school and university and entering
the health professions. Aboriginal and Islander health professionals and health
workers are highly valued in Australian Health and Social Services for their ability
to bridge both worlds. However, the shadows of colonisation continue to impact
on workplace relationships, and the supervision relationship requires sensitive
development. Ensuring an inclusive work environment, one that is perceived as
safe, valuing, and supportive of Aboriginal people, requires attention to several
factors, and our story unpacks some of the supervision strategies that may help.

BOX 4.8B

Part 2: Introducing Monica, Charmaine, and Lenny

Monica is a senior manager in a rural university department supervising a range
of health professionals including occupational therapists, social workers, and
nurses. She works closely alongside and supervises Lenny, a health sciences
graduate who works as a community development officer and is also completing
her Master of Social Work degree. Lenny identifies as a Yamaji woman belonging
to the Southern Yamaji group of the Yamaji nation. Charmaine also forms part of
this working alliance and contributes in the context of her leadership and ability
to provide expert review of our work as a senior Aboriginal academic.

BOX 4.8C

Part 3: Factors that maintain Connections within the working and supervisory relationship

When Monica and Lenny reflect on their working relationship, including within
supervision, they identify the following factors that are important in maintaining
their relationship:

Trust and respect

A commitment to invest in a supportive and well-structured relationship is vital. Lenny emphasises that an honest relationship is highly valued. Many Aboriginal people are excellent readers of non-verbal and body language. They can easily identify dissonance between what is being said and what is being communicated non-verbally. If they observe this dissonance, they may not call it out but may instead distance themselves both physically and emotionally from the relationship.

Lenny must feel that she can trust Monica, as she sometimes needs to share sensitive and personal information. Developing trust and respect includes acknowledging the importance of power-sharing in the relationship and that both supervisor and supervisee have knowledge and expertise to bring to the relationship and the organisation. Trust allows for sharing of information that leads to greater understanding of the contexts that influence Aboriginal ways of working, including cultural responsibilities and creating a safe physical and psychological space.

Role clarity

We are both aware that working in community health environments can throw up unexpected and quite varied daily tasks and responsibilities. Having clear expectations of what our professional roles entail, and the scope of practice, is vital.

We have agreed ways to share information with some short regular meetings and longer in-depth meetings less frequently. When we meet, we have an agreed agenda and follow up with emails outlining actions and the confirmed timelines for completion. We both make notes of all discussions and agreements. As we work out and about in the community we use and share our online calendars and use text messaging, so we know where each other is located.

Inevitably in community settings and particularly in community development settings, new opportunities present themselves. When this happens, we meet to discuss our priorities. As a respected member of the local Yamaji community, Lenny is often asked to contribute to new endeavours. Some of these activities align with her community development role and others may be less of a priority for her role. Lenny sometimes must make difficult decisions regarding what she can take on. She relies on the support of her supervisor in evaluating the most effective use of her time and expertise.

Having a 'yarn'

Face-to-face conversation is especially important as a way of building a solid working relationship and exchanging information. Many Aboriginal people have low levels of trust when communicating with non-Aboriginal people, particularly when communicating with white, Anglo-European people. The reasons for this lack of trust relate to the colonisation issues, but these are not just historical.

Aboriginal people in Australia continue to experience racism and generational disadvantage. They are cautious about building deep relationships until they know that they are not being negatively judged. Lenny values the opportunity to talk through issues to ensure that she understands work priorities and what is required of her, and to articulate her work priorities and how the dynamic community context is likely to influence what can be achieved. Aboriginal people call this style of communication '**yarning**'.

While it sounds informal and has informal elements, including the exchange of personal information, it is also an important form of consultation. Yarning helps build trust and overcomes mistrust. The exchange of personal information and checking in on wellbeing comes at the beginning of the yarn, and is an important step before moving to the discussion on work matters. As trust has built between Lenny and Monica over the years the exchange of personal information is often quite brief, and they can quickly move to discussions on work-related matters.

Personal disclosure does not need to be threatening for supervisors if they enter the yarning process with a commitment to **cultural humility** (Greene-Moton and Minkler, 2020). This can be defined as: **"a lifelong commitment to self-evaluation and critique, to redressing power imbalances … and to developing mutually beneficial and non-paternalistic partnerships with communities on behalf of individuals and defined populations"** (Tervalon and Murray-García, 1998, p. 123).

Using a yarning approach in a virtual environment calls for even more intentional communication strategies to build trust and create a safe space. Be prepared to spend more time building the relationship and exchanging information so that the supervisor and supervisee have a sense of connection with each other. Attend to the environment so that you can see each other clearly, know if anybody else is on the meeting, and that everyone is fully briefed on how to use the technology. If possible, share the lands from which you are speaking and check in with the other person what lands they are currently located on. More details on creating a welcoming physical environment in virtual and physical settings are discussed next.

BOX 4.8D

Part 4: Examples of how to adopt a position of cultural humility

Using the examples Monica and Lenny have experienced in their relationship, the next part shares what adopting a position of **cultural humility** looks like in practice.

Cultural awareness and responsiveness

Educating oneself about Aboriginal culture and communities is important for all our work, but particularly so when in a supervisory relationship with an Aboriginal person. In Australia there are over 200 different Aboriginal groups and over 50 different active languages. We must not make assumptions that if we know about one Aboriginal group, we know about all Aboriginal groups. Making time to find out about history, language, art, family structures, local Elders, and decision makers in the community is vital. Asking relevant questions demonstrates genuine interest in the history and experiences of local Aboriginal people. Again, adopting a position of cultural humility is important.

Physical environment

A message of respect and trust is built when we create a physical environment that is welcoming and acknowledges the local Aboriginal communities. Displaying art, the use of local textiles, patterns on uniforms, designs on webpages and official documentation, and incorporating elements of local language, all send a message of respect and valuing of Aboriginal culture. These resources also provide conversation starters and acknowledgement more broadly of the value placed by the organisation on Aboriginal culture.

Most importantly, employing Aboriginal people sends a powerful message that the organisational environment is a safe place. Incorporating workplace protocols for acknowledging traditional owners, for example Acknowledgement of Country statements, reinforces the respect the workplace has for local Aboriginal people and their culture, which creates a safe environment for Aboriginal employees.

Cultural responsibilities: Adding value to the organisation

Aboriginal people have many family and cultural responsibilities related to their positions within their communities and related to their family structure and where they sit or belong. These responsibilities come with obligations that may impact upon work availability. In many Australian workplaces, cultural leave is available for Aboriginal people; however, it is also important that supervisors and supervisees understand the significance of the cultural responsibilities and obligations, as they may place significant emotional as well as time demands on people.

Monica is aware of Lenny's responsibilities and supports her participation in community obligations, as this work evidences her seniority within the community. Recognition of her senior cultural role, for example when Lenny is asked to conduct 'Welcome to Country' events in the community, enhances her profile as a senior and respected Aboriginal person. Monica understands that this recognition of Lenny's seniority within the community also helps enhance her reputation within the workplace and will have a ripple effect on the work she does for the organisation.

Acknowledging the past

Monica knows that every relationship with an Aboriginal and Torres Straits Islander person is touched by the history of colonisation and dispossession experienced by the Aboriginal people of Australia over the past 230 years. Understanding this history, and in particular the intergenerational trauma from the Stolen Generations that continues to impact on the lived experiences of Aboriginal people, requires an ongoing position of cultural humility.

Listening is particularly important. Lenny values a supervisory relationship that is respectful of her and demonstrates empathy. Monica attempts to embed these values in her relationship by acknowledging the past and being honest and open in her communication style, checking in with Lenny if she is unsure about her response to work-related directions.

As a practical way of acknowledging the past, Monica has the following strapline at the end of her emails: "We acknowledge Aboriginal and Torres Strait Islander peoples and communities as the Traditional Custodians of the land we work on and pay our respects to Elders past, present, and emerging. We recognise that their sovereignty was never ceded. We are committed to cultivating inclusive environments for all people. We celebrate, value, and include people of all backgrounds, genders, sexualities, cultures, bodies, and abilities."

BOX 4.8E

Part 5: Recognising knowledge, skills, and experience

Honouring evidence

Both Lenny and Monica, as health professionals, acknowledge the importance of evidence-based practice. This includes, for Monica, a recognition of Aboriginal bodies of knowledge, some of which are preserved orally, and an incorporation of these knowledge bases into her practice. In this situation she learns from Lenny and other Aboriginal health professionals and scholars. The integration of two-way learning and lifelong learning is important for Lenny and Monica as they endeavour to practise in two cultural worlds.

Many Aboriginal people enter health professional careers in adulthood having worked in other areas and/or after occupying carer roles. They bring a wealth of experience and knowledge that may not be reflected in their formal qualifications.

The number of practising Aboriginal health professionals is low and the number in senior roles and leadership positions is very low.

The organisation must be attentive to the importance of mentoring and encouragement, so Aboriginal employees feel supported to participate in ongoing professional development, as well as considering opportunities to move into more senior roles.

BOX 4.8F

Part 6: Take-home messages

While all work-based relationships must be based on mutual respect, supervisors of Aboriginal people need to understand the complex historical and contemporary events that influence the lived experience of Aboriginal employees, value their cultural responsibilities, and acknowledge the additional knowledge and skills they bring to the workplace. It is tempting to argue that these principles apply to all supervisory relationships or to supervisory relationships with employees who are of culturally diverse backgrounds. We believe that the underlying historical and sociopolitical events that changed the lives of Aboriginal and non-Aboriginal people in the past continue to have an influence on us in this place at the time of writing, and that supervisory relationships must acknowledge this reality.

Good practice working as a supervisor with Aboriginal colleagues requires:

- getting to know the history of colonisation from the Aboriginal viewpoint, and the impact of this history on past and current generations
- familiarising yourself with the concept of cultural humility and focusing on developing power-sharing and equalising relationships
- having clear, negotiated expectations of the worker role that acknowledge their cultural commitments
- using shared calendars, agendas, and documented plans for workflow management
- incorporating physical and material resources in the workplace such as Aboriginal art and cultural items to send a message of valuing Aboriginal culture
- exploring new ways of communicating like yarning, to develop relationships built on trust and mutual respect, valuing what Aboriginal employees bring to the organisation, and
- having a broader commitment to increasing the Aboriginal health workforce in organisations so that Aboriginal, First Nations, Indigenous people are part of leadership teams, supervising others and contributing to organisational outcomes.

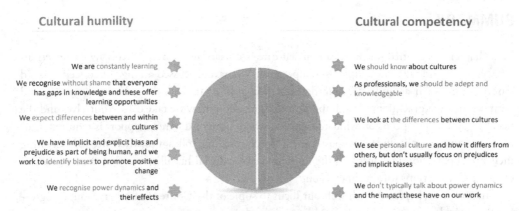

Cultural humility

We are constantly learning

We recognise without shame that everyone has gaps in knowledge and these offer learning opportunities

We expect differences between and within cultures

We have implicit and explicit bias and prejudice as part of being human, and we work to identify biases to promote positive change

We recognise power dynamics and their effects

Cultural competency

We should know about cultures

As professionals, we should be adept and knowledgeable

We look at the differences between cultures

We see personal culture and how it differs from others, but don't usually focus on prejudices and implicit biases

We don't typically talk about power dynamics and the impact these have on our work

FIGURE 4.5 Differences between cultural humility and cultural competence (adapted from Agner, 2020)

Once you have read this reflective story a few times, think about it in relation to our previous discussions about creating safe physical and psychological spaces, cultivating holistic development, demonstrating vulnerability, characteristics within the permeable practitioner model, identifying defence mechanisms, and building capacity in others.

One key message that we have taken away from Monica, Lenny, and Charmaine's reflective story is the concept of cultural humility. Currently our profession talks more about cultural competence as a marker of good practice. We would like to acknowledge the differences between cultural competence and cultural humility (see **Figure 4.5**, adapted from Agner, 2020). We feel we are beginning to see a maturity within the profession and a shift towards cultural humility but appreciate there is still much work for us to do.

CRITICAL COMMENTARY

Finding it difficult to look after ourselves in the helping and caring professions

From our experiences and from the conversations we continue to have with friends and colleagues, it seems that it is often those of us who work in the helping and caring professions who find it particularly difficult to look after ourselves, to show our vulnerabilities, and to ask for help. Before we jump to the conclusion that it is somehow part of our DNA and simply who we are (adopting a fixed mindset), we need to explore the organisational and societal narratives in which we work. For example, in some countries, there is an unhelpful portrayal of health and care workers as superheroes. This has been especially evident in the response to the global pandemic. But this places unrealistic expectations on us and potentially dehumanises practitioners at a point when asking for help and being human is what is really needed to take care of ourselves. Perhaps it is time for us as professionals to own our vulnerabilities, just like the rest of society, as part of connecting with and taking care of ourselves to support others.

Our hope is that you will revisit some of the concepts within this chapter at moments when the superhero cape is either in the cupboard, or when you feel you are being made to wear it when you would rather not. It is in these moments we can take a breath and think about how we wish to respond, to be kind to ourselves, and to be good enough.

SUMMARY

This chapter has centred on the idea that self-care is a relational concept involving Connections with yourself and with your supervisor/supervisee. We have discussed a range of concepts to aid Connections, such as understanding defence mechanisms, unhelpful or destructive roles, and permeability as a practitioner. It is important to think about how we take care of ourselves and the needs of others in supervision while recognising when more or different support is required. Our role as a supervisor includes signposting, e.g. to counselling colleagues when needed. Creating inclusive supervision practices and the importance of cultural humility are vital components to enhance Connections within supervision.

In our next chapter, we will shift our focus to some of the **Content** of supervision, recognising the interplay between the relationships and the doing of the supervision work.

REFERENCES

Agner, J. (2020) 'Moving from cultural competence to cultural humility in occupational therapy: a paradigm shift', *American Journal of Occupational Therapy*, 74(4), pp. 1–7. doi:10.5014/ajot.2020.038067.

Brown, B. (2010) *The power of vulnerability: TEDxHouston*. Available at: https://youtu.be/X4Qm9cGRub0 (Accessed: 20 December 2021).

Brown, R., Desai, S., and Elliott, C. (2020) *Identity-conscious supervision in student affairs*. Abingdon: Routledge.

Choy, A. (1990) 'The winner's triangle', *Transactional Analysis Journal*, 20(1), pp. 40–46. doi:10.1177/036215379002000105.

Greene-Moton, E. and Minkler, M. (2020) 'Cultural competence or cultural humility? Moving beyond the debate', *Health Promotion Practice*, 21(1), pp. 142–145. doi:10.1177/1524839919884912.

Harding, D. (2019) 'Practitioner permeability and the resolution of practice uncertainties: a grounded theoretical perspective of supervision for allied health professionals'. PhD thesis. University of London. Available at: https://eprints.kingston.ac.uk/id/eprint/43854/ (Accessed: 10 July 2021).

Harding, D. (2021) *Ideas and resources for supervision*. Available at: https://thepermeablepractitioner.com/ideas-and-resources/ideas-and-resources-for-supervision/ (Accessed: 10 July 2021).

Health Education England (2020) *Workplace supervision for advanced clinical practice: an integrated multi-professional approach for practitioner development*. Available at: www.hee.nhs.uk/our-work/advanced-practice/reports-publications/workplace-supervision-advanced-clinical-practice (Accessed: 10 July 2021).

Karpman, S. (1968) 'Fairy tales and script drama analysis', *Transactional Analysis Bulletin*, 26(7), pp. 39–43. Available at: www.karpmandramatriangle.com/pdf/DramaTriangle.pdf (Accessed: 7 November 2020).

Lemma, A. (2016) *Introduction to the practice of psychoanalytic psychotherapy*. Chichester: Wiley Blackwell.

Malan, D. (1995 [1979]) *Individual psychotherapy and the science of psychodynamics*. 2nd edn. Oxford: Butterworth-Heinemann.

Shohet, R. and Shohet, J. (2020) *In love with supervision: creating transformative conversations*. Monmouth: PCCS Books.

Tervalon, M. and Murray-García, J. (1998) 'Cultural humility versus cultural competence: a critical distinction in defining physician training outcomes in multicultural education', *Journal of Health Care for the Poor and Underserved*, 9(2), pp. 117–125. doi:10.1353/hpu.2010.0233.

Wilson, A., McCallum, C.M., and Shupp, M.R. (2019) *Inclusive supervision in student affairs*. Abingdon: Routledge.

CHAPTER 5

Organising the content of supervision

Joanne M. Baird, Jodie Copley, Karina Dancza, and Priya Martin

With contributions from Shamala Thilarajah and Wendy H. Ducat

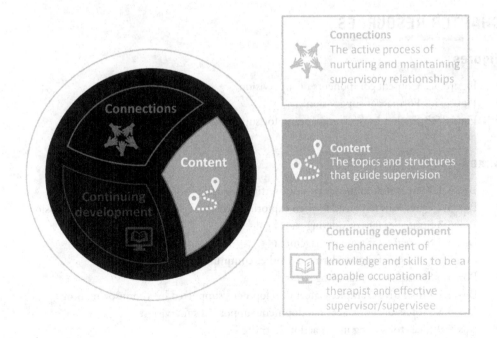

Connections
The active process of nurturing and maintaining supervisory relationships

Content
The topics and structures that guide supervision

Continuing development
The enhancement of knowledge and skills to be a capable occupational therapist and effective supervisor/supervisee

DOI: 10.4324/9781003092544-5

CHAPTER INTENTIONS

In this chapter, we invite you to:

- Explore focal areas for supervision Content
- Consider the practicalities of supervision
- Decide on ways you would like to arrange, plan, and conclude supervision.

CHAPTER HIGHLIGHTS

- Focal areas and topics for supervision Content (direct practice skills and decision making, supporting theory-to-practice connections, professional skills, career planning)
- Practical considerations for supervision Content (format, location, frequency, and duration)
- Session-by-session planning (arranging supervision, initial supervision sessions, ongoing supervision sessions, concluding supervision)
- Critical commentary: Are supervisory agreements a help or a hindrance?

CHAPTER RESOURCES

Figures

- Figure 5.1 Content components of supervision
- Figure 5.2 Formats of supervision
- Figure 5.3 Session-by-session planning for supervision

Boxes

- Box 5.1 Factors that influence priority-setting in supervision
- Box 5.2 Questions to consider when exploring skills and decision making in supervision
- Box 5.3 Strategies for considering workload
- Box 5.4 Strategies for time management
- Box 5.5 Strategies for considering coworker communication
- Box 5.6 Strategies for managing stress
- Box 5.7 Illustrative example: Career development supported by a sponsor/mentor
- Box 5.8 Professional or career development support in supervision
- Box 5.9 Ideas for setting up an action learning set
- Box 5.10 Quality telesupervision characteristics
- Box 5.11 Questions to consider when finding a space for supervision
- Box 5.12 Four essential elements of a supervision arrangement/agreement/contract
- Box 5.13 Guiding questions for the supervisor to get the first supervision meeting started
- Box 5.14 Typical supervision documentation

- Box 5.15 Practical tips for monitoring and evaluating supervision
- Box 5.16 Questions to consider when concluding supervision

Appendices

- Appendix 5.1 Content of supervision preparation sheet
- Appendix 5.2 Supervision agreement template
- Appendix 5.3 Supervision session record

THE CONTENT OF SUPERVISION

This chapter will explore what we mean by **Content** within the 3Cs of Effective Supervision. Content covers the **focus, topic, and details covered in supervision; practical considerations that structure supervision (e.g. format, location, frequency, and duration of supervision); and session-by-session planning of supervision**.

Figure 5.1 illustrates the co-creation of this Content between the supervisor and supervisee. The illustration also indicates different components that we will discuss here, but there is room for additional components such as those related to **Connections** discussed in Chapter 4 and **Continuing development** in Chapter 6. We will start by considering potential focus and topic areas for supervision before moving on to the practical details of setting up the sessions and session-by-session planning. We invite you to look at the Content preparation sheet in **Appendix 5.1**, as this offers a summary of key areas and prompts for crafting the Content of supervision.

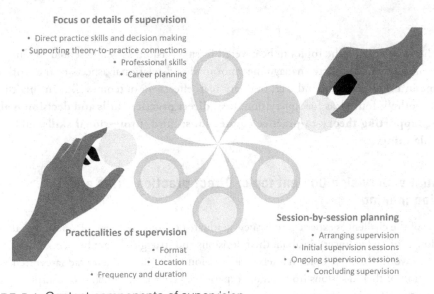

Focus or details of supervision
- Direct practice skills and decision making
- Supporting theory-to-practice connections
- Professional skills
- Career planning

Practicalities of supervision
- Format
- Location
- Frequency and duration

Session-by-session planning
- Arranging supervision
- Initial supervision sessions
- Ongoing supervision sessions
- Concluding supervision

FIGURE 5.1 Content components of supervision

FOCAL AREAS AND TOPICS FOR SUPERVISION CONTENT

Supervisors, supervisees, and the organisation you work for will likely have an opinion about what to focus on during supervision. Thus, the focus of supervision is something that is likely to require negotiation. There may be **specific local or national guidelines** that need to be followed in some contexts, as we discussed in Chapter 1. In other circumstances, there is a need to prioritise what topics to address, so that supervision can be specifically targeted, and the supervisee is not overwhelmed. This decision begins with a full appreciation of what there is to learn in the specific workplace and role, with some ideas presented in **Box 5.1**.

BOX 5.1

Factors that influence priority-setting in supervision

The focus of supervision may be influenced by the:

- **core business** of the organisation or work unit
- **key responsibilities of the supervisee** within their role and how this interacts with the bigger picture of service provision
- **perspectives of the supervisee** regarding skills or practices they feel more or less confident about, and
- **perspectives of the supervisor, or other colleagues' observations or feedback** regarding priorities for the supervisee's development (informally or through appraisal processes).

When considering the topics to be covered in supervision, as we presented in Chapter 4, the importance of support to manage the emotional and relational aspects of the work must be borne in mind given the indirect, but very real, effects on outcomes. But in this chapter, we will spotlight four ideas for supervision: first, **direct practice skills and decision making**; second, **supporting theory-to-practice connections**; third, **professional skills**; and finally, **career planning**.

Potential supervision Content topic: Direct practice skills and decision making

A review of the challenges experienced by new graduate occupational therapists found that novice practitioners often felt uncertain about their decisions and struggled to apply their knowledge and skills when working with people on interventions (Moir et al., 2021). New graduates often sought confirmation of their decisions from a more experienced colleague, which is not surprising given the complex and varied information they need to integrate to plan person-centred interventions (Copley et al., 2010).

In a situation where skill development and decision making are prioritised, a first step might be to **define the key knowledge, skills, and competencies required** in the practice area. In some larger organisations, competency frameworks that detail these skills will have already been developed (Turpin et al., 2021). If not, spend some time deciding these (perhaps with reference to national standards offered by professional associations or other bodies) so that there is full consideration of what is needed to practice in this area and a plan can be negotiated, agreeing on suitable areas to prioritise in supervision. A note of caution here is **not to try to reinvent your own framework** for each job role. From our own experience, we have found creating 'homegrown' tools extremely time-consuming, difficult to obtain consensus, and the product is unlikely to be recognised outside your organisation without rigorous evaluation. Our perspective is to start with established guidance and adapt it to your specific situation, such as the Career Development Framework developed in the United Kingdom by the Royal College of Occupational Therapists (RCOT, 2021; see also Chapter 2).

When learning something new, **people require time and repetition**. When it is a complex skill, such as making decisions about assessment and intervention approaches, more time and effort are required than when learning technical skills and following established procedures. Experienced supervisees are also likely to benefit from a focus on how decisions are made as the complexities of the role also increase over time, making integration of knowledge, skills, and professional judgement an ongoing area for development. Ideas for how to address this Content area in supervision can be drawn from chapters 1 and 2 where we considered concepts such as supervision models and learning and teaching principles. Chapter 6 also provides tools for the supervisor as we discuss how to provide feedback and promote reflection. For now, **Box 5.2** highlights some questions that guide the **Content** of supervision sessions when the focus is on direct skills and decision making.

BOX 5.2
___

Questions to consider when exploring skills and decision making in supervision

- Is there **knowledge** underpinning the skills that needs to be revised or sought out through **accessing educational opportunities**?
- Have I had **exposure to the practice of more experienced colleagues** through discussing examples, observing their practice, or having access to intervention plans and reports? If not, could I ask for this to happen?
- How can I keep a record of the **principles of practice**, 'rules of thumb', and **decision-making cues** I notice in the practice of others?
- What techniques can I use for **reflection in and on practice**, during and after sessions?
- Could creating a **visual representation of more experienced therapists' decision making** in practice (e.g. a flowchart, a diagram, etc.) help me to develop my understanding of my own reasoning?

- If I mapped out the **occupational therapy process** with a person accessing my services in mind, could I explain and justify the connections between my assessment, intervention, and evaluation strategies?
- What **evidence** can I gather regarding the **quality of my practice** (from the people I work with, evaluation tools, etc.)?
- What **professional models** or frameworks have I considered? Are there others that could give me a different perspective?

Potential supervision Content topic: Supporting theory-to-practice connections

Another common topic or focus for supervision is linking theory with practice. Using a **professional model or framework** in supervision, as a foundation to discuss skills and knowledge, can help clarify the roles and responsibilities that an occupational therapist is expected to fulfil.

Using the occupational therapy process as the foundation for discussion (e.g. the Occupational Therapy Intervention Process Model (OTIPM) (Fisher, 2009; Fisher and Marterella, 2019), then expanding on each step with complementary profession-specific or related knowledge, offers a consistent structure for approaching theory-to-practice connections. For example, when goal setting, Self-Determination Theory could be useful to understand a person's motivation for change that guides interventions (Poulsen et al., 2015). Using the occupational therapy process as a consistent framework enables the specific tasks carried out by a therapist (e.g. assessments and interventions) to be explicitly linked together and connected with the bigger picture to support occupational performance and participation. For more details about using the occupational therapy process to frame practice, please see Dancza and Rodger (2018).

Supporting theory-to-practice connections is a vital and valuable part of supervision. But it is not always easy to do for a range of reasons. Sometimes when people have considerable experience, they work more intuitively and may not always explain how theory informs their practice to a supervisee. It is also possible that some occupational therapists are clear about a theory or perspective they follow but may be reluctant to critique it or feel uncomfortable if others do not hold the same views. Whatever the case, raising theory as a topic for discussion in supervision in a way that both supervisee and supervisor feel comfortable is important so you can unpack your role and articulate a clear professional basis for your practice. You could find this safe space in any part of your portfolio of supervision (see Chapter 3).

Potential supervision Content topic: Professional skills

The efficiency and effectiveness of practice is often underpinned by one's professional skills – **workload, time management and prioritisation, coworker communication, and self-management (including stress management)**. Such skills are arguably more difficult to learn than professional practice or technical skills, and so may need to be an intentional focus in supervision, particularly given their critical role in enabling high-quality outcomes in service provision.

Early career occupational therapists cite challenges in meeting all their work-related responsibilities by balancing direct work with people with other tasks such as documentation, preparation, team meetings, etc. (Moir et al., 2021). **Box 5.3** illustrates some strategies for considering **workload**.

BOX 5.3

Strategies for considering workload

- **Understand the full extent of your workload** by mapping out all tasks in the role and the current time allocation for each. Discuss with your supervisor if the time allocation could or should be redistributed.
- Create a list of tasks that make up a typical week or month. Highlight what you **need to do** (e.g. the number of people you are required to see) and **want to do** (e.g. interest groups, committees). Discuss if you think there is a balance between these to allow both meeting responsibilities and maintaining motivation. If you feel you are overcommitted with what you need to do, can you raise the idea in supervision to create a long-term plan to fit in desired roles gradually over time?

Finding your pace of work and keeping up with expectations, particularly when entering a new workplace, can be another challenge. Arguably it remains a challenge as you become established in your career when more opportunities may present themselves. There are various **time management** strategies that you can try as you settle into your role, and a few ideas are suggested in **Box 5.4**. We gently encourage you to practise the art of saying no to some of the 'opportunities' that are presented to you, or ensuring that the ones you say yes to are those that align with your career goals.

BOX 5.4

Strategies for time management

- Seek out **time management or prioritisation tools and techniques** to optimise efficiency, for example, organising and reprioritising one's tasks at the beginning of each day, prioritising the top three tasks to be completed each day or scheduling in protected time for all non-contact related tasks (e.g. documentation).

- Break down the time spent on different tasks this week and put them on a chart; what does it look like? To what extent does this match what an ideal or successful use of time might be?
- Determine whether **templates, proformas, or exemplars** for common tasks such as therapy planning and reports are available, or could be created, to save time and provide structure and guidance.

Another reported difficulty for early career occupational therapists is working in interprofessional teams, as well as communicating with colleagues within their own professions in some workplace cultures (Moir et al., 2021; Murray et al., 2020). **Box 5.5** offers some ideas for **developing coworker communication**. These are also of value to established professionals when starting a job within a new organisation or sector.

BOX 5.5

Strategies for considering coworker communication

- **Locate role models** within the workplace who are working productively in teams. What is it that they are doing well? Can you arrange a time to talk with them about how they approach working in a team?
- **Reflect on your communication experiences** when you have had a conversation with a team member, using a reflective tool such as the Model of Professional Thinking (see Chapter 6). This can help you to unpack what happened and learn for next time.

When workload, time management, coworker communication, or many other factors are not ideal, it can lead to stress. **Stress** is a natural part of life and something which can be helpful for productivity in the right amount. Too much stress, however, is counterproductive and can impact not only work, but personal life and health as well. Monitoring your stress levels and seeking support from your supervisor or others if you feel it is getting out of hand is important throughout your working life. **Box 5.6** offers a few ideas to help with stress, although there are many other strategies available in self-help guides, phone applications, etc. We have also discussed some ideas in relation to self-care in Chapter 4.

Potential supervision Content topic: Professional development (career) planning

Professional development or career planning is another potential focus for supervision and may be particularly relevant when supervising mid-career or senior occupational therapists (although it could be a conversation at any career stage). Career planning involves assisting the

BOX 5.6

Strategies for managing stress

- What **stress management strategies** do you use already? For example, how do you balance work, leisure activities, and rest? Do you use strategies or tools such as deep breathing techniques or phone applications that could also help at work?
- Would you like to find **professional development opportunities** to further develop skills to manage stress (e.g. growth mindset or mindfulness)?
- What are your own personal and professional values? How are these reinforced or challenged within your workplace? What can you do to find a balance between the way you like to work and the way you need to work?
- If possible, discuss with your supervisor what their perspectives are on how much is enough in relation to the quality and quantity of work completed. Does it match with yours? Do you need to **recalibrate your expectations and self-judgement**?

supervisee to plan their career direction and the steps they might take to get there. It may also include an element of **sponsorship**. Sponsorship is where the supervisor helps to promote the supervisee's career by providing networking opportunities (Rothwell et al., 2019), connecting them with key people in the field and perhaps inviting them to work on the supervisor's own projects.

A focus on career planning is likely to share similarities with mentoring, with the supervisor providing advice based on their own experience and facilitating the supervisee's passage into a new professional sphere. We offer an illustrative example (**Box 5.7**) where an experienced health professional shares how valuable and necessary he found having a sponsor and mentor to further develop his career.

BOX 5.7

Illustrative example: Career development supported by a sponsor/mentor

As an experienced health professional, I have spent 15 years in practice and the past four years in a specialist area while I completed my PhD. I found it challenging to return to a full-time role working directly with people who access services after my studies. I had developed new knowledge and skills during my PhD, and I was keen to put them into practice, but existing service structures and my position in the organisation were somewhat limiting. While my existing supervisor tried to help,

I found that as they were not a subject matter expert, they were less able to guide me to maximise what I could do within my existing job scope.

I was extremely fortunate that at around the same time the head of the department nominated me for the organisation's mentoring programme. I was asked to choose mentors from a list, and I selected people from outside my profession as I wanted a broader perspective on my role.

I was glad when I got my first choice and set up my first meeting with my mentor. Within a few sessions, my mentor already understood my perceived limitations in what I was able to do in my current role. My mentor also encouraged me to see the way around it. Helpfully, they also created opportunities for me to present my work on different platforms, thus helping to build my reputation as an expert. My career took off!

I am extremely grateful for access to the mentoring programme. I still value my regular supervision as they offer me practical support such as allocated time and day-to-day help. But it was my mentor's encouragement and the opportunities they created for new adventures that has enabled me to work to my full potential.

This illustrative example highlights how helpful it can be for an experienced person (who is probably also a supervisor) to consider their own supervisory needs. It may be that you are at a point in your own career where you, like the health professional in the example, could benefit from expanding your own supervisory portfolio (as introduced in Chapter 3) to include mentorship/sponsorship. **Box 5.8** offers a few ideas about what career development Content in supervision discussions might look like, and you can think of these from the perspective of a supervisor and/or supervisee.

BOX 5.8

Professional or career development support in supervision

- Take stock of your established skills and the most satisfying components of your work role.
- Explore **options to engage in new activities or seek a new position**, either within the current organisation or another workplace, that would allow application and growth of skills.
- **Think about the four pillars of practice in the Career Development Framework:** professional practice, leadership, facilitation of learning, and evidence research and development (RCOT, 2021). Which pillar(s) would you like to enhance in your existing role?

- **Define the steps** needed to make this move, remaining **positive** about your capacity and potential to take on a new, more senior, or challenging role.
- Consider where you might **look for a sponsor or mentor**. Think about formal or informal opportunities within and outside of your organisation or profession (see also Chapter 9).

The focus topics within supervision are not static, and it is likely that you will be working on more than one area at a time. Being responsive to changing needs and situations, even from session to session, may be required. In this next section, we will shift the conversation to the practical structures for supervision as these will create opportunities for you to address the priority focal areas.

PRACTICAL CONSIDERATIONS FOR SUPERVISION CONTENT

How supervision is delivered depends on the needs of the supervisee and is also influenced by the supervisor and context of the setting. We will start by describing a few **different formats or general supervisory approaches** that can be considered as stand-alone methods, or more likely in combination as you create your portfolio of supervision.

Format of supervision

We can think about the format of supervision in terms of:

- **how formal or informal** the supervisory arrangements are (e.g. mandated time, catch ups when needed)
- **who is involved** (e.g. one or more supervisors and supervisees, peers, people from different professions, etc.), and
- **how it takes place** (e.g. in-person, at a distance using technology, while travelling together, etc.)

Figure 5.2 outlines some common formats of supervision. While all formats have their merits (and challenges), we will discuss two here in more detail – action learning sets and telesupervision.

Action learning sets

Action learning is an approach to development, both at the individual and the organisational level, that has been applied to healthcare for many years (Edmonstone, 2018). It is suited to healthcare because it is particularly helpful in addressing 'wicked' problems, that is, the complex, multidimensional, and context-dependent issues that are encountered daily in the professional practice that occupational therapists typically do.

Action learning is like group supervision (which we explore in Chapter 7), as it involves people coming together in regular 'set' meetings. It also shares some commonalities with Communities

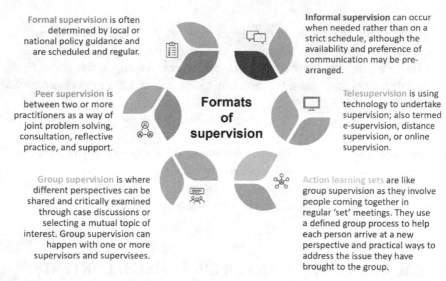

FIGURE 5.2 Formats of supervision

of Practice (Barbour et al., 2018; Barry et al., 2017) and Balint Groups (Sargeant and Au-Yong, 2020). Action learning uses a defined group process to help each person arrive at a new perspective and practical ways to address the issue they have brought to the group. In essence, action learning sets help you to see your issue or problem through fresh eyes, allowing you to generate possible solutions or actions that were not previously visible. **Box 5.9** outlines common features of successful action learning sets (Haith and Whittingham, 2012).

BOX 5.9

Ideas for setting up an action learning set (adapted from Haith and Whittingham, 2012)

- A regular (closed) group of approximately three to seven people
- Meetings supported by management and prioritised by members
- Ongoing and regular meetings, such as every four to six weeks
- Agreed time limits for each sharing and subsequent discussion, such as 30–60 minutes per person
- Turn taking happens so that all members contribute to presenting and facilitating issues
- Confidentiality arrangements for discussions are in place
- Members do not offer solutions to the presenter of the issue; they ask questions to bring aspects of the issue into the presenter's awareness
- Meetings typically are facilitated by a regular person (who could be the supervisor) who does not present their own issues

Telesupervision

Historically, face-to-face supervision has been the most common type and perhaps even your own preferred style. However, the use of telesupervision is on the rise. Telesupervision uses technology to undertake supervision which could be on a computer, mobile device, telephone, etc. It is also termed e-supervision, distance supervision, online supervision, and perhaps has other names too.

Telesupervision has been used in rural and remote areas for many years, where distance and service structures mean that supervisees and supervisors are not in the same location. Telesupervision has been used in other situations for convenience, but its use has been accelerated by the global COVID-19 pandemic and our increased reliance on technology to remain connected with others when physical proximity is undesirable. Any of the previously described formats of supervision could be conducted using telesupervision, but may require some adjustments to maintain effectiveness.

We anticipate that with the increasing reliance on technology to support working practices, research into the effectiveness of telesupervision may also expand in the coming years. However, at the present time, research on telesupervision in the post-registration phase remains sparse. Based predominantly on the findings of a systematic review (Martin et al., 2018) and the authors' collective experience with facilitating telesupervision arrangements for health professionals over many years, we have consolidated some characteristics of quality telesupervision in **Box 5.10**.

BOX 5.10

Quality telesupervision characteristics

- Having a **supervision arrangement** with clear expectations of all parties
- Thorough **preparation** including finding a quiet space, preparing and sending out an agenda prior to the session, testing the equipment and connectivity
- Well-structured sessions with a **clear agenda**
- Outline of topics/cases and **expected contributions** of people present, prior to the session
- **Flexibility (and calmness!)** to manage delays due to technical issues
- Careful **record keeping** using supervision minutes that can be referred to after the session and as a recap in the following session
- The length and timing of meeting needs to be tailored to the number of people present, supervisee's stage of career, learning needs, etc. **Shorter and more frequent sessions** may be preferred as online concentration may be different from face-to-face meetings

---

There is evidence to show that some face-to-face contact, especially before using telesupervision or in the early stages of the supervision partnership, is beneficial (Martin et al., 2018). This could be the result of the supervisor and supervisee(s) already being familiar with each other's communication style and a possible pre-established mutual trust and respect. Where previous face-to-face contact has not been possible, frequent supervision sessions are recommended in the initial stages of telesupervision to establish the partnership. Seeking opportunities to supplement virtual presence with a physical presence, such as at a meeting or conference is another strategy to enhance telesupervision relationships.

Once the format for supervision has been discussed, it is also important for the location to match the requirements of the session. We will explore this in the next section.

Location for supervision

Supervision time is precious and needs to be valued by both the supervisor and supervisee, and supported by the workplace management. Therefore, finding a confidential, quiet location, free from interruptions, where both supervisor and supervisee can speak freely, is important. Turning off distractions such as phones, computers, or messaging applications indicates that attention is focused on the supervision tasks. Some have suggested that supervision being held away from the workplace is beneficial as supervisees feel more supported to reflect on complex situations or share sensitive issues more freely (Martin et al., 2014). **Box 5.11** outlines some questions to ask when finding a space for supervision.

BOX 5.11

Questions to consider when finding a space for supervision

- Have you pre-planned and agreed on the venue?
- Is the venue comfortable, confidential, and away from the supervisee's work unit?
- Can you make the supervision venue distraction-free? Can you use 'do not disturb' signs on the door and turn your phones off while the session is in progress?
- Is the location of supervision convenient and practical? For example, at times it may be appropriate have supervision take place during an interaction with a person accessing services to provide 'hands-on' feedback, or where notes are stored to facilitate document review.

Finding the right space is equally important when using **telesupervision**. Issues commonly reported are background noise, audio lags, use of old or incorrect equipment, and supervisee/supervisor lack of competence and confidence in operating videoconference equipment. Additional time may need to be allocated before sessions to set up equipment and troubleshoot issues. However, recognising that even the most technologically savvy person will have days when systems have problems can help you to remain calm and make other arrangements, rather than becoming overwhelmed and frustrated (which is what we find is often our go-to response!).

If **supervising in a group**, we have found it helpful if all participants are either online in their own separate space, or all in the same room for a face-to-face session. Issues often arise when there is a hybrid of people in the room and online (unless you are using specific videoconferencing facilities with suitable microphones, etc.). For example, if more than one computer is used in the same room there is often an issue with audio feedback, or people who are not directly in front of the computer are not heard by those online. When all participants are online, everyone has the same access to information and sharing, it helps reduce side-conversations which can exclude people.

Frequency and duration of supervision

Supervision frequency and duration may be mandated or guided by local or national supervision policies. Often these guidelines recommend minimum requirements for supervision to be met by employers. These guidelines are often minimum standards rather than optimal requirements.

The frequency and duration of supervision may differ according to the seniority level of the supervisee, how long a person has been in a role, and the availability of other support (e.g. peers or more experienced colleagues) in the setting. **People who are new to a role, new in their career, or working in isolated situations (e.g. as a lone practitioner) are likely to require more frequent and longer supervision sessions** (Martin et al., 2014). Clear guidelines for how often and how long supervision should happen are perhaps more commonly seen with student or new graduate supervision. When there is no clear policy, it is up to the supervisor and supervisee (along with any relevant management input) to determine what is needed.

Experts in professional supervision have noted that sessions should be regular, with some recommending **sessions every four weeks** (Butterworth, 1997), although more may be needed for early career, isolated, or newly appointed therapists. One study found that health professionals who received supervision for at least 45 minutes monthly were more satisfied that their supervision was effective than those who received less. For less experienced supervisees, more than this minimum was needed (Snowdon, 2018). Other studies recommend **between one and two hours per session**, which provides enough time for in-depth discussions and/or observations, but not so much as to overwhelm the supervisee with feedback (Winstanley and White, 2003; Edwards et al., 2005).

SESSION-BY-SESSION PLANNING

We have discussed in this chapter the focal areas for supervision content and practicalities of supervision. In our final section on the Content of supervision, we propose and discuss four broad time periods along the supervision journey: (1) arranging supervision, (2) initial supervision sessions, (3) ongoing supervision sessions, and (4) concluding supervision, as illustrated in **Figure 5.3**.

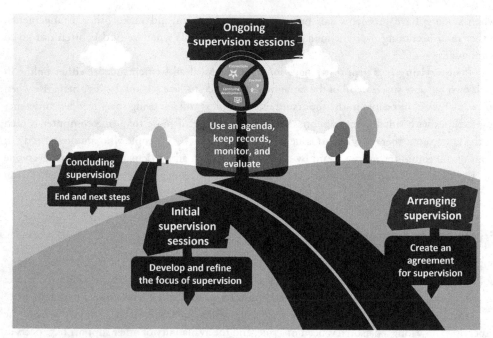

FIGURE 5.3 Session-by-session planning for supervision

Arranging supervision

Supervision can be viewed as a journey for the supervisor and supervisee. Because supervision is for a specific purpose and period of time, agreeing what will happen is a key task when arranging supervision. A **supervision arrangement** acknowledges that supervision is a process – a working relationship – that is different from other work relationships.

We see a supervision arrangement as a **mutually agreed and helpful discussion (rather than the paperwork that captures it) to clarify roles and expectations**. In your setting or circumstance a **formal contract** may be appropriate if, for example, there is payment involved or there are legal protections needed. We encourage you to seek advice locally so you can make an informed decision. However, we acknowledge that there are times when the relationship between supervisor and supervisee may benefit from more **organic development**. In this case it may be that a conversation about expectations is sufficient, or that plans are made along the way.

A supervision arrangement specifies the structure of the supervisory relationship as well as what is to be learned or gained. The arrangement is a way to acknowledge the rights and responsibilities of each person and sets the stage for clarity moving forward to support a positive outcome (Martin et al., 2014). The format of the **arrangement may be verbal or written**. When making this decision we invite you to think about the pros and cons of both formats. For example, a verbal arrangement could set an informal tone for the supervision, help develop rapport between parties and remain flexible to the evolving working relationship. Having a written agreement helps reduce the potential for miscommunication, offers a clear prompt that can be reviewed, can acknowledge the value placed on supervision, and may be helpful if concerns arise later in the working relationship (Yeung et al., 2001).

Box 5.12 outlines four essential elements of the supervision arrangement, and if you do not have a specific format within your organisation, Appendix 5.2 provides a template that can be adapted to meet your requirements.

BOX 5.12

Four essential elements of a supervision arrangement/agreement/contract

- **Type of supervision** – Will it be one-on-one, a form of a group supervision model, face-to-face, telesupervision, or a combination of all?
- **Rights and responsibilities of the supervisor and the supervisee** – How will the relationship be defined? Set specific ground rules for what the expectations are and how they will be met. Ensure attention is paid to managerial, educative, and supportive functions of supervision.
- **Goals and objectives of the supervision itself** – Ultimately, what is the aim of this endeavour? How will each party know that this aim has been fulfilled? What is the timeframe for these goals and objectives?
- **Working arrangements** – These are the activities both parties agree to do. What are the expectations for supervision sessions, documentation, and communication systems, opportunities provided, and the evaluation process that will be used to determine progress? What is the process if tensions arise in supervision and how will supervisors and supervisees access independent support?

Initial supervision sessions

Once supervision is arranged, the initial supervision meetings will probably involve further discussions about the focal areas for supervision content and any refinements to the structure of the sessions. This discussion fosters Connections (as discussed in Chapter 4), collaboration, and provides a foundation for the working relationship (Yeung et al., 2001). The way you approach these initial meetings will differ depending on the situation and where the supervisee is in their career. You may wish to review the novice to expert continuum introduced in Chapter 2 along with considering the guiding questions in Box 5.13 to get the meeting started.

Ongoing supervision sessions

The Content of supervision refers to both the topics and details that are discussed, and the structures that frame and support these discussions. When supervision is ongoing, the topics will evolve based on the priorities of the supervisee and any external influences from the work being undertaken. To frame and support these supervisory discussions, it can be helpful to establish

BOX 5.13

Guiding questions for the supervisor to get the first supervision meeting started

Share information about professional experience, past and present:
- What would you like to tell me about your current role/work?
- What would you like to know about me?

Discuss the expectations and aims of supervision:
- What would you like to gain/attain from this?
- What working arrangements did you have in mind?

Discuss previous experience of supervision:
- Have you had any previous experiences with supervision?
- How was this conducted? How well did it work for you?

Discuss any anxieties about the process:
- What are your expectations for these sessions?
- What are your concerns?
- [If appropriate] I know that you have been assigned to me as a supervisor/ supervisee, rather than having made this as a free choice. Does this raise any concerns or anxieties for you?

Ask about the priority topics that the supervisee wishes to discuss:
- Do you have any topics, situations, cases that are a priority for you right now and you would like to discuss?
- Tell me more about what you have been working on recently.
- Talk me through what you have been doing in the past week.

routines such as using an agenda for supervision, keeping track of sessions using a documentation format, and continuously monitoring and evaluating supervision.

Using an agenda for the supervision session

Although a clear agenda or schedule is typically considered a characteristic of all effective professional meetings, when we think of the varied functions of supervision (learning, support, feedback, validation, etc.), it is worth considering the possible benefits and limitations of having an agenda for each session.

In terms of benefits, **an agenda will assist accountability**, ensuring that the time is used in a directed way rather than subsumed by general or unrelated discussion, particularly if the supervisor and supervisee work in the same unit. It can also legitimise the supervision session as in some situations, meetings are cancelled if there is no agenda, assuming people have nothing to discuss.

However, at times the **task-focused nature of a tight agenda could be limiting**. Understanding the supervisee's practice and exploring issues deeply (as in action learning) or creating a vision of where they want to be (if using appreciative, strengths-based approaches) may require free discussion of the supervisee's context, expression of emotions and frustrations, and exploration of new possibilities. It is therefore advisable that, for at least some supervision sessions, **flexibility is applied in following an agenda** so that important discoveries are not glossed over, and people feel comfortable in raising insights or observations that occur in the moment.

When an agenda is used, it is often recommended that this be set by the supervisee, to foster ownership and responsibility for directing the supervision, as well as a sense of control. Again, there are some caveats. For example, supervisees who are underperforming **may selectively avoid addressing issues or may not be aware of gaps in their knowledge or skills** (Rothwell et al., 2019). This lack of awareness or avoidance may not be apparent to the supervisor as they have access only to information the supervisee provides, rather than the whole picture. Considering these potential pitfalls, it is recommended that, particularly early in the supervision arrangement, the supervisor asks **the supervisee to recount their practice in a narrative way** (e.g. 'Tell me about that session you had yesterday,' or 'Talk me through what happened in the team meeting,' or 'Break down for me how you went about that data search'). Such accounts of practice help the supervisor to detect potential issues that require exploration but have thus far remained invisible to the supervisee. Effective supervision often involves a touch of detective work!

The next element that is likely to require some attention is how you will keep track of sessions and what documentation you think will assist with this, and we will consider this next.

Keeping track of sessions

Supervision documentation typically consists of a supervision arrangement (please see earlier discussion), agenda, notes, and logs (see **Box 5.14**). Supervision documentation needs to be stored confidentially and maintained well as it may serve as legal evidence should a matter be taken up in performance management or legal proceedings.

BOX 5.14

Typical supervision documentation

- Supervision agendas outline what is going to be covered in a session
- Supervision log is a record of the supervision date, time, duration and may also contain brief notes on the various topics discussed in the sessions. Sometimes, these logs are helpful for department heads who may audit supervision practices to ensure compliance with organisational professional support or supervision policies
- Supervision notes are detailed notes of the discussions that occurred in the supervision sessions. It is good practice for the supervisor and supervisee to decide on who takes notes and how they will be stored etc.

- Reflective logs can be based on a reflective model and allow supervisees space to capture learning and reflections in advance so it can be discussed in depth within the supervision session (see Chapter 6).

The documentation requirements vary depending on your employing organisation and/or registration bodies. If you do not have an existing structure or want to update what you already use, there is a template for a supervision session record that you could adapt in **Appendix 5.3**. Keeping track of sessions is an ongoing process and is likely to also include monitoring and evaluation, which we will explore in the next section.

Monitoring and evaluating supervision

Supervision monitoring and evaluation can be both formal and informal. While evaluation may occur at most stages of a supervision process, periodic formal reviews can be useful to ensure it is still meeting people's needs, to renegotiate terms, or to end the arrangement.

Informal evaluation may include a review of the outcomes of supervision. For example, the supervisee and supervisor could discuss the outcomes for people who access the services provided by the organisation, or progress made on the development of specific skills and techniques (**Continuing development**). Informal review could also include adherence to professional standards and ethics (**Content**). There should also be a focus on the process of supervision and if the activities and format are meeting the needs of the supervisory relationship (**Connection**) (Martin et al., 2014). Towards the end of each supervision session, it could be as simple as the supervisor asking, "Has this session provided what you need today?".

While informal and regular 'touching base' is important to keep supervision on track and correct immediate issues, **formal evaluation** too has a role in tracking overall quality of the arrangement. Formal evaluation methods could include focus group interviews, semi-structured interviews, or self-report questionnaires (see Chapter 9 for a list of commonly used supervision evaluation tools). These formal evaluation methods could also form part of any supervision research or audits at a work unit, department, or organisation. As a starting point for considering how to monitor and evaluate supervision, we invite you to reflect on the points made in **Box 5.15**.

BOX 5.15

Practical tips for monitoring and evaluating supervision

- Use a combination of informal and formal methods to evaluate supervision.
- Build supervision evaluation into the supervision arrangement.
- Review supervision documentation to construct your feedback for the supervision evaluation.

- Review the learning needs of the supervisee, how they are being met, or how they have evolved.
- Review the focus and practicalities of supervision sessions and if they are still appropriate.
- Review the format of supervision (e.g. face-to-face, telesupervision, etc.) and consider if it is still appropriate.
- If you are using telesupervision, consider if the mode of technology you use is still suitable or if there is a better platform that can be tried.
- Invite feedback on your performance, both as a supervisee and a supervisor. This may come from those involved directly within your supervisory relationship, peers, and/or other managers or supervisors who are familiar with your work.
- Remain open to receiving feedback and acting on it.
- Consider how the style of supervision is helpful (or not).

Monitoring and evaluating supervision can help the relationship remain productive and effective, but there will be a time when supervision ends, and that is the focus of our final section.

Concluding supervision

The supervisory relationship will eventually end, and thinking about how this will happen at the beginning can help ensure all parties are prepared. We need to **start supervision with the end in mind**.

In some cases, supervision will be a defined number of sessions, perhaps because there is payment involved. For other cases, there may be a set period of supervision defined by a regulatory body, such as a 12-month period for new graduates. In these cases, it will be clear when the supervisory relationship will end or be renegotiated. In other situations, the supervisory relationship may be more open-ended as the positions held by the supervisor and supervisee dictate the arrangement; for example, supervision may only conclude when either party leaves the job. In any case, it may be useful at the start of the relationship to discuss how it will end, or at least when it will be reviewed if there is no clear end point.

If you have developed a written supervision arrangement at the start of your relationship, this could be a useful document to review when concluding supervision. You may also wish to revisit any learning objectives created or other markers of what you originally wanted to achieve from supervision (we will explore learning objectives in Chapter 6). **Box 5.16** offers some additional questions to consider when ending a supervisory relationship. If you feel that supervision has not met your expectations or it has not gone as well as you hoped (as either the supervisor or supervisee), you may also benefit from raising these issues with someone you trust. Further ideas for how to manage tensions in supervision are discussed in Chapter 8.

> ### BOX 5.16
>
> ### Questions to consider when concluding supervision
>
> - Did you gain what you wanted? If not, what are your next steps?
> - Is there another arrangement needed? Do you need to look for something elsewhere?
> - Does the relationship need to change into something else, such as a peer or mentor relationship?
> - To what extent did you complete the tasks of a supervisor or supervisee?
> - What worked? What could you do differently next time?
> - Do you need a break from this relationship or form of supervision?
> - Did this relationship end abruptly? If there is something unfinished, how can you transition to something else?

CRITICAL COMMENTARY

Are supervisory agreements a help or a hindrance?

Our reading of current research into supervision seems to point to the positives of using a supervisory agreement or contract when formulating supervision. We have, however, had long discussions about the impact of designing the content of supervision in a very procedural way. For example, when we work with people who access our services, our initial approach is to use our relationship to support progression, and we may only use a formal agreement if something is not going according to plan (unless it is a contract for a paid service). Similarly, there is a risk that a contract or agreement introduced early on could make the supervisory relationship feel unduly formal, as in some settings people are only put on a 'contract' if they are being performance-managed because they are not performing to minimum standards.

To share another example that we debated; although we like to think that supervision is always a positive experience, we also know there can be a darker side to it. Callahan and Watkins (2018) highlight that supervision can be poor-quality, ineffective, and even harmful, including emotionally abusive encounters that can impact on the supervisee's functioning and work. In one study of harm in supervision, Ellis et al. (2014) reported that many supervisees had harmful supervision in the past. While we don't like to think about it, it does remind us that supervision can be the source of workplace problems. A written supervisory agreement could perhaps mitigate harmful supervision, but due to the inherent power imbalances in supervision, we wonder if it would really be enough if someone is intent on being manipulative and causing harm.

Finally, we considered the current research basis for supervision and wondered if we don't yet know enough to draw a conclusion about the effects of a supervisory agreement or contract. Maybe it is related to the experience and comfort of the supervisor in guiding the relationship, or to the context of the organisation, or something else? While this would make an interesting study, in the meantime it makes sense to use our own judgement of the situation (just like we do when working with people who access our services) to formulate the topics and shape the structures of our supervisory relationships. That is why we have deliberately chosen to use the phrase 'supervisory arrangement', so it remains flexible to meet different contexts. What we feel is of importance is the need to invest time to agree and make arrangements to ensure that supervision is prioritised in busy work settings so, if an agreement or contract helps to create this dedicated time and space, it is of value, even in a brief format. We can use tools as we have suggested in the appendices as a starting point, but we would not want supervision to be a rigid procedure that sacrifices the all-important supervisory relationship.

SUMMARY

Supervision has a different purpose from other workplace relationships, and therefore it is beneficial to consider how supervision time is used to best effect. The Content of supervision in the 3Cs for Effective Supervision includes focal areas for supervision topics and the structures that help us frame these discussions. The **Content** of supervision may be the most tangible of the three parts to our framework so is perhaps a useful place to start. However, keep in mind the importance of **Connections** as previously explored, and the next chapter, **Continuing development**, as all three components are needed for effective supervision.

REFERENCES

Barbour, L., Armstrong, R., Condron, P., and Palermo, C. (2018) 'Communities of practice to improve public health outcomes: a systematic review', *Journal of Knowledge Management*, 22(2), pp. 326–343. doi:10.1108/JKM-03-2017-0111.

Barry, M., Kuijer-Siebelink, W., Nieuwenhuis, L., and Scherpbier-de Haan, N. (2017) 'Communities of practice: a means to support occupational therapists' continuing professional development: a literature review', *Australian Occupational Therapy Journal*, 64, pp. 185–193. doi:10.1111/1440-1630.12334.

Butterworth, T. (1997) *It is good to talk: an evaluation of clinical supervision and mentorship in England and Scotland*. Manchester: School of Nursing, Midwifery and Health Visiting, University of Manchester.

Callahan, J.L., & Watkins, C.E., Jr. (2018) 'The science of training III: supervision, competency, and internship training', *Training and Education in Professional Psychology*, 12(4), pp. 245–261. doi:10.1037/tep0000208.

Copley, J.A., Turpin, M.J., and King, T.L. (2010) 'Information used by an expert paediatric occupational therapist when making clinical decisions', *Canadian Journal of Occupational Therapy*, 77, pp. 249–256. doi:10.2182/cjot.2010.77.4.7.

Dancza, K.M. and Rodger, S. (eds) (2018) *Implementing occupation-centred practice: a guide for occupational therapy practice learning*. Abingdon: Routledge.

Edmonstone, J. (2018) 'Conferences as sites of learning and development: using participatory action learning and action research approaches', *Action Learning: Research and Practice*, 15(2), pp. 193–197. doi:10.1080/14767333.2018.1464747.

Edwards, D., Cooper, L., Burnard, P., Hanningan, B., Adams, J., Fothergill, A., and Coyle, D. (2005) 'Factors influencing the effectiveness of clinical supervision', *Journal of Psychiatric and Mental Health Nursing*, 12(4), pp. 405–414. doi:10.1111/j.1365-2850.2005.00851.x.

Ellis, M.V., Berger, L., Hanus, A.E., Ayala, E.E., Swords, B.A., and Siembor, M. (2014) 'Inadequate and harmful clinical supervision: testing a revised framework and assessing occurrence', *The Counseling Psychologist*, 42(4), pp. 434–472. doi:10.1177/0011000013508656.

Fisher, A.G. (2009) *Occupational therapy intervention process model: a model for planning and implementing top-down, client-centered, and occupation-based interventions*. Fort Collins, CO: Three Star Press.

Fisher, A.G. and Marterella, A. (2019) *Powerful practice: a model for authentic occupational therapy*. Fort Collins, CO: Center for Innovative OT Solutions.

Haith, M.P. and Whittingham, K.A. (2012) 'How to use action learning sets to support nurses', *Nursing Times*, 108(18–19), pp. 12–14.

Martin, P., Copley, J., and Tyack, Z. (2014) 'Twelve tips for effective clinical supervision based on a narrative literature review and expert, *Medical Teacher*, 36(3), pp. 201–207. doi:10.3109/0142159X.2013.852166.

Martin, P., Lizarondo, L., and Kumar, S. (2018) 'A systematic review of the factors that influence the quality and effectiveness of telesupervision for health professionals', *Journal of Telemedicine and Telecare*, 24(4), pp. 271–281. doi:10.1177/1357633X17698868.

Moir, E.M., Turpin, M.J., and Copley, J.A. (2021) 'The clinical challenges experienced by new graduate occupational therapists: a matrix review', *Canadian Journal of Occupational Therapy*, 88(3), pp. 200–213. doi:10.1177/00084174211022880.

Murray, C.M., Edwards, I., Jones, M., and Turpin, M. (2020) 'Learning thresholds for early career occupational therapists: a grounded theory of learning-to-practise', *British Journal of Occupational Therapy*, 83(7), pp. 469–482. doi:10.1177/0308022619876842.

Poulsen, A., Ziviani, J., and Cuskelly, M. (2015) 'The science of goal setting', in Poulsen, A., Ziviani, J., and Cuskelly, M. (eds) *Goal setting and motivation in therapy: engaging children and parents*. London: Jessica Kingsley Publishers, pp. 28–39.

Rothwell, C., Kehoe, A., Farook, S., and Illing, J. (2019) *The characteristics of effective clinical and peer supervision in the workplace: a rapid evidence review*. Newcastle: Newcastle University.

Royal College of Occupational Therapists (2021) *The career development framework: guiding principles for occupational therapy*. London: Royal College of Occupational Therapists. Available at: www.rcot.co.uk/publications/career-development-framework (Accessed: 31 August 2021).

Sargeant, R. and Au-Yong, A. (2020) 'Balint groups for foundation and GP trainees', *British Journal of Psychotherapy*, 36, pp. 481–496. doi:10.1111/bjp.12562.

Snowdon, D.A. (2018) 'Clinical supervision of allied health professionals'. PhD thesis. La Trobe University.

Turpin, M., Fitzgerald, C., Copley, J., Laracy, S., and Lewis, B. (2021) 'Experiences of and support for the transition to practice of newly graduated occupational therapists undertaking a hospital graduate program', *Australian Occupational Therapy Journal*, 68(1), pp. 12–20. doi:10.1111/1440-1630.12693.

Winstanley, J. and White, E. (2003) 'Clinical supervision: models, measures and best practice', *Nurse Researcher*, 10(4), pp. 7–38.

Yeung, E., Jones, A., and Webb, C. (2001) 'The use of learning contracts', in Kember, D. (ed.) *Reflective teaching and learning in the health professions: action research in professional education*. Oxford: Blackwell, pp. 68–83.

Appendix 5.1: Content of supervision preparation sheet

FOCUS OF SUPERVISION
The priorities for the supervisee(s) currently are (tick all that apply and provide details):
☐ Practice skills and decision making: ☐ Theory-to-practice connections: ☐ Professional skills: ☐ Career planning: ☐ Other:
FORMAT OF SUPERVISION
The initial format for supervision will be (tick all that apply and provide details):
☐ Formal (specify who will be involved): ☐ Informal (specify what is acceptable e.g. email, messaging, etc.): ☐ Peer (specify who will be involved): ☐ Group/action learning sets/other: ☐ Telesupervision:

LOCATION OF SUPERVISION

Supervision will happen (specify location):
Location will be arranged/booked by (name of person):
Confidentiality will be ensured by (list measures):
Distractions will be minimised by (list measures):

FREQUENCY AND DURATION

Guidelines applicable to this situation state (list requirements):

The frequency of supervision will be (daily /weekly/monthly, etc.):

The duration of each session will be (30/60/90 minutes, etc.):

The sessions will be planned for the following period (1/3/6/12 months, etc.):

The process if the session needs to be changed is (list how and when):

ARRANGING SUPERVISION

An arrangement for supervision has been developed (tick and provide details):

☐ **Yes** (state if it is written or verbal):
☐ **No** (specify how expectations will be made clear):

Supportive functions of supervision are recognised in an arrangement (tick and provide details):

☐ **Yes** (state what this will look like):
☐ **No** (state how the supervisee will seek support):

There is a process in place for seeking alternative support (for supervisor or supervisee):

☐ **Yes** (state what this is):
☐ **No** (state how any concerns can be raised):

INITIAL SUPERVISION SESSIONS

Note key areas or questions you intend to cover in your first few sessions (tick and make notes or create your own)**:**

☐ Sharing information about past and current professional experience:
☐ Expectations and aims of supervision:
☐ Previous experiences of supervision:
☐ Any anxieties about the process:

ONGOING SUPERVISION SESSIONS

An agenda for supervision has been developed (tick and provide details):

☐ **Yes** (list the format and who is responsible for its completion):
☐ **No** (specify how expectations will be made clear):

Supervision documentation formats have been developed (tick and provide details):

☐ **Yes** (list the format, storage, and who is responsible for its completion):
☐ **No** (specify how sessions will be recorded):

Monitoring and evaluation of supervision will include (tick all that apply and provide details):

☐ Monitoring questions (provide examples and when this will happen):
☐ Review of supervision arrangement (note how and when this will happen):
☐ Review of learning objectives (note how and when this will happen):
☐ Review of focus of supervision (note how and when this will happen):
☐ Review the practicalities of supervision (note how and when this will happen):
☐ Use evaluation questionnaire(s) (note what tools and when this will happen):
☐ Others will be involved in the monitoring and evaluation (note who, how, and when):

CONCLUDING SUPERVISION
This supervisory relationship intends to end (tick and provide details): ☐ At a fixed date (note the date): ☐ After a set number of sessions (note the number of sessions): ☐ After achievement of an objective (e.g. full registration, completion of a project): ☐ It is open-ended (note when it will be reviewed):

Appendix 5.2: Supervision agreement template

This template offers an initial structure for preparing a supervision agreement and is intended to be tailored based on your own context and modified as your supervisory relationship evolves. It is written in a practical way rather than a legal manner so please check local requirements to ensure this meets your needs. This template has been adapted from: Substance Abuse and Mental Health Services Administration (US), 2009; Cassedy, 2010.

THIS DOCUMENT SERVES AS A WORKING AGREEMENT TO DESCRIBE THE SUPERVISION PROVIDED BY:
Supervisor (name, position, employer): to Supervisee (name, position, employer):
DATE OF AGREEMENT
DATE OF REVIEW
PRACTICALITIES Format: Location: Frequency: Duration: Scheduling/cancelations/attendance:
COSTS, IF APPLICABLE
FOCUS OF SUPERVISION The focus of supervision has three broad functions: formative, normative, and supportive: • **Formative/educative:** supporting the development of skills to promote the 'doing' of tasks • **Normative/managerial:** supporting caseload and workplace management • **Restorative/supportive:** support monitoring and recognition of the stressors involved in a task, situation, or environment Specific areas/topics/goals that will or will not be included in this supervisory relationship are:

SUPERVISION DOCUMENTATION AND MONITORING
• [Form name] will be used to document the content and progress of the supervision sessions • Informal feedback will be provided (time and how): • Formal feedback will be provided at the end of each session (how): • Written formal evaluation will be provided [frequency] about [progression toward goals, aims, objectives; satisfaction with supervisory process] • Supervision notes will be shared (when, how, with whom):
DUTIES AND RESPONSIBILITIES
The supervisor at a minimum will [please amend as needed]: • Prepare for the supervision session by minimising distractions, ensuring no interruptions, reviewing prior session information. • Be reliable; prioritise sessions; maintain time boundaries, confidentiality, and agreement terms. • Offer supervision 'first aid' for current urgent/emergent concerns/issues. • Encourage the supervisee to seek outside support or advice when necessary and assist to facilitate access to this support. • Challenge any behaviour, action, or reasoning that the supervisee displays or discusses which raises concern about their practice, development, use of supervision, or which could be hurtful to others. • Reflect on own supervisory skills and ensure that there is support for the supervisor themselves (e.g., a support system/own supervision). • Present and model appropriate professional practices and behaviours. • Ensure that ethical guidelines and legal statutes are upheld. • Monitor progress, and work with external agents or resources as appropriate and agreed. • Request and remain open to feedback about own supervisory performance. [add any additional duties or responsibilities as needed]
The supervisee at a minimum will [please amend as needed]: • Prepare for supervision by identifying discussion items. • Attend the formal supervision sessions. • Give the supervisory relationship a high priority by arriving punctually. • Be prepared for the discussion by eliminating other distractions. • Ask for assistance or support to develop and progress toward goals, objectives, and targets. • Commit to professional development by making and then following through action plans. • Be open to constructive challenge and feedback from the supervisor by explaining or justifying actions, and not to interpret appropriate challenge as personal attacks or discriminatory practice. • Provide feedback to the supervisor about what is effective and what is less helpful. • Stay on task and use time to reflect in depth, while avoiding non-productive conversation. • Uphold all ethical guidelines and legal statutes. • Consult supervisor or designated entity in emergencies. • Implement reasonable supervisor directives. • Adhere to all appropriate policies and procedures. [add any additional duties or responsibilities as needed]
PROCEDURAL CONSIDERATION
• Any development plan/goals and objectives will be discussed and amended if necessary. • The quality of the supervisory relationship will be discussed, and conflicts resolved. • If conflicts cannot be resolved, [name and contact details] will be consulted. • Crises or emergency consultations will be documented. • Due process procedures (as explained in the employing organisation's policy and procedure handbook) have been reviewed and will be discussed as needed. • Confidentiality of supervisory discussions will be maintained unless any disclosure is agreed, or there is concern for the safety of the supervisee/supervisor or others.

This agreement is subject to revision at any time upon request of either person. Revision will be made only when mutually agreed. We agree to uphold the directives outlined in this agreement to the best of our ability and to conduct our professional behaviour according to the ethical principles and codes of conduct of our professions.

Supervisor_____   Title_____   Date_____

Supervisee_____   Title_____   Date_____

Appendix 5.3: Supervision session record

Date, time, format, and location of session	
Persons present (supervisor/supervisee/peer(s)/guest)	
AGENDA / TOPICS TO DISCUSS	DISCUSSION / NOTES
Action items/outcomes	
Signatures	
Next session details	

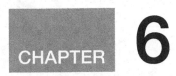

Preparing for supervision and continuing the development of your supervisory skills

Jodie Copley, Joanne M. Baird, and Karina Dancza

With contributions from Priya Martin, Kyrin Liong, Áine O'Dea, Sarah Harvey, and Stephanie Tempest

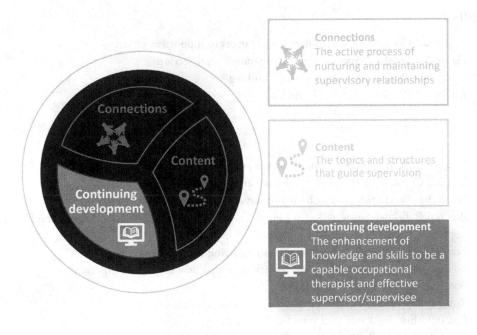

Connections
The active process of nurturing and maintaining supervisory relationships

Content
The topics and structures that guide supervision

Continuing development
The enhancement of knowledge and skills to be a capable occupational therapist and effective supervisor/supervisee

DOI: 10.4324/9781003092544-6

CHAPTER INTENTIONS

In this chapter, we invite you to:

- Explore how to prepare to be a supervisee or supervisor
- Consider how to start working as a new supervisor or supervisee
- Plan and create meaningful learning goals and objectives in supervision
- Review skills in reflective practice and apply them in supervision
- Analyse selected skills necessary for being a supervisor and supervisee.

CHAPTER HIGHLIGHTS

- Preparing to be a supervisee or supervisor
- Creating learning goals and objectives
- Reflection in supervision
- Active listening and effective questioning
- Giving and receiving feedback
- Critical commentary: Are SMART goals a bad idea?

CHAPTER RESOURCES

Figures

- Figure 6.1 Goals to learning objectives to targets to supportive actions
- Figure 6.2 Levels of learning that are dependent on reflection
- Figure 6.3 The Model of Professional Thinking
- Figure 6.4 Pendleton Feedback Model

Boxes

- Box 6.1 Reflecting on prior experiences of supervision
- Box 6.2 Considering the practicalities of being a supervisor
- Box 6.3 Reflecting on your skills as a supervisor
- Box 6.4 Reflective Story by Kyrin Liong: Cross-disciplinary supervision and feeling like an imposter
- Box 6.5 Topics to consider in preparation for being a supervisee
- Box 6.6 Questions to consider when working with a new supervisee/supervisor
- Box 6.7 Starting points for reflection
- Box 6.8 Editor's Reflective Story: Learning through reflection
- Box 6.9 Thinking about your own levels of learning
- Box 6.10 Editor's Reflective Story: Using the Model of Professional Thinking

- Box 6.11 Effective listening principles
- Box 6.12 Techniques for enhancing communication in telesupervision
- Box 6.13 Reflective Story by Áine O'Dea: The power of listening to the supervisee
- Box 6.14 Reflective Story by Kyrin Liong: Supportive feedback that relied on developing the working relationship
- Box 6.15 Characteristics of useful feedback

Appendices

- Appendix 6.1 Creating learning goals and objectives guidance template
- Appendix 6.2 Model of Professional Thinking guidance template
- Appendix 6.3 Pendleton feedback guidance template

PREPARING TO BE A SUPERVISEE OR SUPERVISOR

Within the 3Cs for Effective Supervision, we have discussed **Connections** in Chapter 4 and **Content** in Chapter 5, bringing us to the final component, **Continuing development**. This refers to two aspects, **(1) development as an occupational therapist (whatever role you may be in), and (2) development as a supervisee or supervisor**. In this chapter, we will be referring to both aspects but emphasising professional development as a supervisor and supervisee, as this is the focus of our book and something that, in our opinion, has not received as much attention.

As occupational therapists, we have many skills that enable us to design and conduct interventions and interactions. However, **being a supervisor to professional colleagues is quite a different pursuit that requires us to adapt and add new skills to our tool kit**. In fact, there is substantial evidence from health profession research that **supervisors should receive specific education in supervision skills** (Rothwell et al., 2019). It is not uncommon for supervisors to adopt supervision strategies and techniques that we ourselves have experienced throughout our professional careers. This can offer a useful starting point; however, we want to be intentional and take only the best of what we have experienced and let go of less helpful practices. Consider the questions in **Box 6.1** to help you think about what you would ideally like (or wish to avoid) as a supervisor.

BOX 6.1

Reflecting on prior experiences of supervision

Think about the supervisors you have had, and ask yourself the following questions:

- What does the best supervision look like for you?
- What does the worst supervision look like for you?
- Who was the best supervisor?

- Who was the worst?
- What contributed to those feelings?
- What worked well and why?
- What didn't work and why?

It is also important to consider the longevity and gravity of being a supervisor and how this role fits within the responsibilities you already hold. There may be potential role conflicts, such as:

- If you are a **line manager**, you will need to be mindful of judging the supervisees' ability to do the job properly as they talk about their anxiety when working with a person accessing services or when they discuss a time when they felt that their session had gone badly.
- If you are a very **experienced practitioner**, you may need to monitor how you make suggestions to your supervisees or share what you would have done in their situation. Instead, it is helpful to sit with their exploration of the problem and give people time to come up with their own ideas.
- If you are an occupational therapist offering supervision to a **mixed group of professionals**, you may need to be conscious of any hidden alliances you feel to the other 'like-minded' professionals in the room because they look and sound familiar to you.

Box 6.2 invites you to consider some of the practical elements associated with being a supervisor and potential actions you might take.

BOX 6.2

Considering the practicalities of being a supervisor

- What roles do you currently hold within your team? Do you see any potential role conflicts? If so, what could you do to remain aware of these conflicts and seek to minimise their impact?
- Are you able to allocate time in your own supervision sessions to discuss your role and seek your own support?
- Are you able to add the additional time commitments associated with supervision into your diary/calendar/schedule so you can see the true time commitment of this role? Prior to each session, can you allocate time to prepare the physical or online room and read up notes from the previous session?
- Is there time in your plan for the supervisee(s) to arrive, settle, and start?

- During the session, how do you plan on time keeping?
- When and how do you plan on writing up notes of the session and reflecting on what happened?
- When you are scheduled for holidays, who might be able to facilitate the supervision in your absence?

The practicalities of the supervisory role are important, but not the only consideration for taking on this role. The skills you bring to supervision will also impact on its effectiveness. **Box 6.3** offers a few questions to help you reflect on what you personally bring to the supervision process.

BOX 6.3

Reflecting on your skills as a supervisor

- What supervisory experience, leadership, and group work skills can you bring to supervision?
- How confident do you feel with the theories associated with supervision and group work (if you are planning a group supervisory structure)?
- What professional skills/attributes can you bring to supervision?
- How comprehensive is your knowledge of the organisation?
- How will you know you are not an imposter; what would you notice you were doing that would disprove this idea?

The final question in Box 6.3 may come as a surprise. The reason we chose to include thinking about being an 'imposter' is that it is common in new roles to feel unsure about our performance. At times we may even start doubting our skills and abilities to take on this role. Often this is referred to as **imposter syndrome**, a term coined by Clance and Imes (1978) which describes a situation where people find it hard to take credit for their achievements and have a common fear that they are going to be exposed for not knowing what they are doing.

Imposter syndrome can lead to perfectionism and burnout (Bravata et al., 2019) and it is something important to monitor when becoming a supervisor. Seeking your own supervisory support from a supervisor, peer, or mentor is recommended. The **Reflective Story** by Kyrin Liong **(Box 6.4)**, an engineer who has worked collaboratively across disciplines including in health, describes her experiences of feeling like an imposter as she supervised a member of staff from computer science.

Reflective Story by Kyrin Liong: Cross-disciplinary supervision and feeling like an imposter

As an engineer, working across disciplines either in academia or practice is a common occurrence. As a junior myself charged with the responsibility of supervising someone else, this fact does not make the process any easier. In my very first role as an engineering supervisor to an employee from the computer science department, the experience was both illuminating and terrifying.

The project began well enough, with an idea to use artificial intelligence software to aid in the engineering design process. This required collaboration with a computer science colleague, who brought along with him his junior employee (we will call him Sam). Not long after the commencement though, it was mainly Sam who was working on the project, with me as his day-to-day supervisor. I was incredibly excited for the project but, unfortunately, as the project entered its second phase and more sophisticated programming was involved, I found myself further and further out of my depth. Sam would come to our weekly update meetings and present the critical problems that needed creative computer science solutions. There were a few instances in which, as someone outside his discipline, I offered a fresh perspective that led to a usable solution, but those were few and far between. For the most part, I was left feeling like a 'bad' supervisor for not being able to contribute adequately. I was worried that Sam would feel alone, with seemingly no one he could turn to for guidance.

Eventually, as Sam and I progressed through the project, we found our way and the results were significant enough that we were able to obtain funding to properly study the problem. As I reflected on how we developed our cross-disciplinary working relationship, I realised that there were three key practices that helped strengthen our bond:

(a) **We worked hard to develop a similar language**. I was careful to listen to the technical terms he was using and was unashamed to ask him to clarify any confusions. To facilitate Sam's understanding of the engineering problem, I highlighted a few key terms that he should take note of and did my best to explain them to him. Minimising our communication barrier not only helped us understand each other better, but more importantly, helped the project move forward steadily.

(b) **We often visited each other's departments**. Though a seemingly small gesture, this gave us an opportunity to be immersed in each other's culture, and, even if only for a while, to have a sense of how different things may be. I believe what was valuable in these visits, other than the discussions, was the ability to observe how Sam interacted with his peers, and vice versa. From these observations, I saw that Sam's colleagues operate very similarly to how engineers operate. Recognising this similarity helped me to relax and open up to Sam and that definitely helped develop our working relationship.

(c) Lastly, but perhaps most importantly, **we were patient with each other and let the collegial relationship develop in its own time**. We allowed ourselves the time to learn to speak the other's language, and to learn each other's culture. I firmly believe that, as we did not force or push each other to understand our discipline's language and culture but came from a place of respect and curiosity to truly comprehend, we were able to build collegial trust and a strong foundation upon which our project was successful.

Kyrin's reflections and desire to keep learning and evolving as a supervisor contributed to the ultimate success of her work with Sam. While you may only think about developing skills in supervision when you become a supervisor, professional development in supervision is helpful for both supervisor and supervisee to maximise the effectiveness of your time together.

Professional development to be a supervisee may not be something that is commonly thought about, given that we all start out being supervised, so we might consider it something that will just develop organically. While this could be the case, you can **enhance your experience as a supervisee by investing time to reflect on the purpose of the supervision and what you hope to get out of it** (as discussed in Chapter 5). To help you think about your supervisee role, we invite you to make some notes in response to the questions in **Box 6.5** and discuss them with your supervisor to help establish this relationship and clarify your expectations of supervision.

BOX 6.5

Topics to consider in preparation for being a supervisee

- What are your expectations for the supervisory relationship?
- What specific areas of your development do you want to focus on initially?
- How do you learn? What strategies have you used successfully in the past? What was the situation or context where these strategies worked? Would you like to expand your learning techniques through discussion with your supervisor?
- What motivates you?
- How do you respond when you receive feedback? How do you use feedback to improve your practice, skills, knowledge, or abilities?
- What do you see are your responsibilities for your actions, professional development, and wellbeing? What do you see are the responsibilities of your supervisor in these areas?

For both supervisor and supervisee, the start of any new working relationship can be an exciting experience. There may, however, also be some anxiety with starting something unknown. To help you prepare for the initial supervision session, you may like to reflect on the guiding questions in **Box 6.6**.

BOX 6.6

Questions to consider when working with a new supervisee/supervisor

- What do I know about the supervisee/supervisor I will work with?
- How does what I know about the other person impact on this new relationship?
- Considering what I know, is there any additional preparation I need to do to get the most out of this supervision?
- Will the available supervision resources meet my needs?
- Who can I talk to when I am challenged in my work with this supervisee/ supervisor?

When undertaking the tasks of a supervisor or supervisee, there are some core skills that offer a foundation for effective supervision. While not an exhaustive list, we will focus on the skills of creating learning goals and objectives, reflective practice, active listening, effective questioning, and giving and receiving feedback, in the following sections. We have discussed these in a way that we hope is helpful for both supervisor and supervisee, and these sections could be explored together in supervision.

CREATING LEARNING GOALS AND OBJECTIVES

We are familiar with the need to track progress in our work with people who access our services through the setting of goals and use of outcome measures. Similar principles can be applied to our own development in supervision. **Creating goals and objectives is a shared responsibility of the supervisor and supervisee**. The supervisee can self-assess for areas of strength and areas of growth and begin the process of identifying goals. The supervisor may contribute by specifying general areas of focus, or in some cases, may provide precise ideas as they guide the development of the supervisee. **Figure 6.1** provides an illustration of how a goal can be explored by co-developing learning objectives, targets, and supportive actions for a supervisee named Nhungi.

Goals need to be meaningful to the supervisee. As such, it is helpful for the supervisee to use words that make sense to them (rather than using a prescribed formula). Goals could be developed from the supervisee's understanding of the situation. But it is likely that the supervisor will also guide them to areas that are a current priority from the understanding they gain about the supervisee's skills and performance and the organisation they work in.

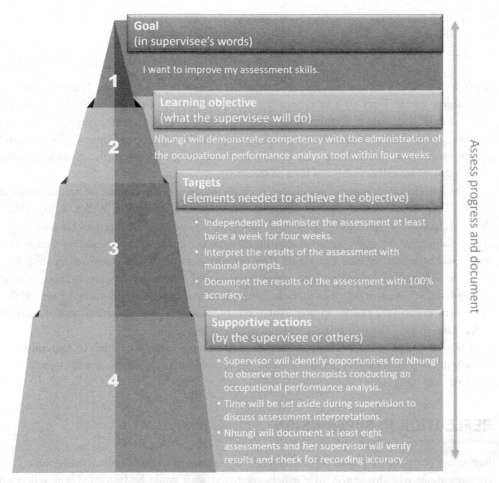

FIGURE 6.1 Goals to learning objectives to targets to supportive actions (adapted from Moran and Dancza, 2018)

From the goal, the idea is to **co-create a learning objective**. This is a clear statement of what it would look like if the supervisee were to achieve the goal (i.e. what would the supervisee be doing differently? How would you know a change has happened? What would you notice?).

To make professional development more obvious and outcomes apparent to all, consider establishing behavioural **targets in tandem with learning objectives**. Partnering learning objectives with targets provides a way to measure progress and growth. While there are multiple methods to do this, one is to begin with the acronym SMART-ER:

- Specific
- Measurable
- Achievable (appropriate to developmental stage)
- Realistic (relevant to professional aims)

- Time-based
- Evaluated
- Recorded

The use of SMART-ER reminds both the supervisor and supervisee that the learning objective and targets should focus on a behaviour, indicate the conditions under which this behaviour is performed, and include a criterion of what represents acceptable performance (Moran and Dancza, 2018). This can transform vague ideas into a concrete plan (see Figure 6.1, steps 2 and 3). However, if you are considering career development or long-term goals, it may not be possible or desirable to write them with this level of specificity.

The foundation of the pyramid in Figure 6.1 is the **supportive actions** that are needed to ensure success. These are actions and responsibilities that the supervisee or others need to take, to help achieve the targets, objective, and ultimately the goal (see Figure 6.1, step 4). The supportive actions can be created through analysing the steps that are required to meet the targets and considering the supports that would help each step (like what we do when working with people who access our services).

The final part of this process is to **assess progress and document**. Documentation includes any updates, revisions, or deletions to the learning objectives, targets, or supportive actions so that movement towards the goal is captured. There may be more than one goal at a time, but don't try to have too many, as there is a danger that focus will be lost.

As a starting point for developing your own goals we have created a template in **Appendix 6.1**. To help develop ideas for your goals, reflection may be a helpful tool, and this is what we will focus on next.

REFLECTION IN SUPERVISION

Reflection is a personal process of thinking about a situation or topic and drawing some conclusions about what happened, why it happened, and what could be learned. Using reflection is a well-established practice within occupational therapy professional education (e.g. American Occupational Therapy Association, 2020; Gribble and Netto, 2020), and an area that we feel is an important skill for Continuing development in supervision.

While learning styles such as Honey and Mumford (2006) classify some learners as reflectors, and others as activists, theorists, or pragmatists, all occupational therapists are taught the importance of reflecting on practice. This is perhaps wise when we consider that, although people may state a learning preference for how they like information presented to them, evidence on the impact of matching someone's learning style to a method of instruction is sparse (Husmann and O'Loughlin, 2019; Pashler et al., 2008).

While critiques about the validity of using learning styles to inform our educational methods are beyond the scope of this chapter, we acknowledge that reflection may not come naturally to every health professional. This is where supervisors can play a key role. For example, supervisors could introduce reflective models, reflective writing or journaling, and discussion with others (Martin et al., 2014). Peer and group supervision sessions can also provide a great opportunity for supervisees to reflect on their practice. Communities of practice, where people who share a common interest in a subject or concern collaborate over an extended period to discuss ideas, source solutions, and build capacity (Cox, 2005), are also a useful forum to promote professional development through reflection and social learning. We will return to social learning ideas when we discuss group supervision in Chapter 7.

For someone learning to use reflection, selecting a topic worthy of investment of time and effort is an important first step. **Box 6.7** offers some questions that may prompt topics for reflection.

BOX 6.7

Starting points for reflection (adapted from Liebel, 2018)

- Which people in my workplace have drawn my attention? What is it about them that I find interesting? Which people in my workplace tend to escape my notice? Why do I think that is?
- Who in my workplace (people who access services, supervisee/supervisor, or colleagues) do I find it more difficult to get along with, or relate to, or reach? How do I feel about this?
- Did anything surprise me today? What was it? Why did it surprise me?
- What is presenting a challenge for me recently when it comes to my role/my workload/the people who access my service/my colleagues/my knowledge base/my supervisee or supervisor?
- What have I found interesting or curious recently?
- What have I done recently that I am proud of?
- If I had a magic wand and could give myself the insights, knowledge, or skills I need to succeed this week, what would I give myself?
- What tricks or productivity boosts have I discovered lately? What might these tell me about myself or the context where I work?
- Who can help me to identify the things that I don't even know I need to know yet?
- Where am I now in my career? What contributed to me getting to here?
- Where do I want to be? How am I going to get there?

When going on courses, working with more experienced therapists, reading relevant literature, engaging in professional association activities – or anything else that contributes to your professional development – reflection will help make the new ideas relevant and applicable to your work. Essentially, reflection is a key component to learning (Moon, 1999, 2004). Without reflection, we are in danger of going about our work with the mindless routine of doing the same thing over and over again (Carroll, 2010b).

Reflection enables us to change what we do and is the process of turning information and knowledge into wisdom (Carroll, 2010b). Using reflection in supervision enables different perspectives to be shared so that the meanings of events can be created, challenged, or changed. This process of learning can be described in many ways, but we will present it in four levels (adapted from Carroll, 2010a). These are using reflection in supervision to (1) solve a problem, (2) change behaviour, (3) change thinking, and (4) change the thinking behind the thinking (**Figure 6.2**). These levels of reflection are illustrated by the **Editor's Reflective Story**: Learning through reflection (**Box 6.8**).

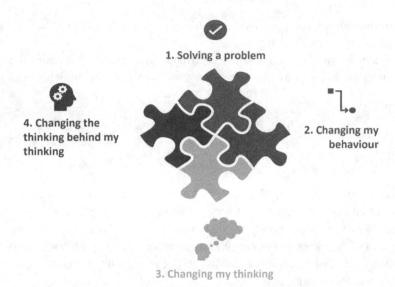

FIGURE 6.2 Levels of learning that are dependent on reflection (adapted from Carroll, 2010a)

BOX 6.8

Editor's reflective story: Learning through reflection

I (Steph) view the levels of learning as situational rather than hierarchical, and I don't think they are levels that you have to work through in a step-by-step way. When I think about my own career so far, I recognise times when I've needed supervisory support and reflection purely to solve a problem but not to explore the issues in more depth, recognising that not every piece of learning requires in-depth meta-analysis if it is essentially a routine challenge.

Equally, I can recall moments within supervision when the light bulb has gone on quickly and shone brightly. In those moments, whether it be from sessions as part of my PhD supervision, managerial supervision, or professional supervision, I have experienced genuine transformational learning where the thinking behind my thinking has been challenged and changed. This has enabled me to discover new worlds of possibilities.

Carroll (2010a) argues the benefits of changing the thinking behind the thinking extends beyond the impact on the individual; once a therapist can embrace new ways of thinking, this creates space and opportunities for new voices to be heard. These include "the quiet, unspoken voices, the powerless voices, the underprivileged voices, the abused voices, the hurt voices" (Carroll, 2010a, p. 16). When we open ourselves up to new voices, then the true power and benefit of learning through reflection in supervision can be realised. If you would like to read more about changing the thinking behind the thinking, we can suggest Transformational Learning Theory and a subset of this in threshold concepts literature. This has been applied in occupational therapy predominately around student learning (e.g. Rodger et al., 2015; Nicola-Richmond et al., 2019; Kaelin and Dancza, 2019), but it is also useful when considering learning after graduation. **Box 6.9** suggests some reflective questions to help you apply the idea of levels of learning to your own practice and perhaps think about your own story.

BOX 6.9

Thinking about your own levels of learning

- Take a few moments to think about a professional experience where you made a change in your thinking. Can you link that experience to a level of learning? How do you know this?
- Can you think of other experiences that can be linked to each level of learning? Or can you recall one experience that addresses several levels?
- What was it that helped you learn in that experience?

We will now turn our attention to how we can support reflective practice with a practical tool. The Model of Professional Thinking (Bannigan and Moores, 2009) proposes a way to connect reflection with evidence-based practice; two vital areas for occupational therapists. The model draws from the common stages of reflective practice identified by Atkins and Murphy (1993), 'what?', 'so what?', and 'now what?', and embeds evidence-based practice in the 'so what?' stage. We have developed our own version of the model in **Figure 6.3** but encourage you also to read the original article (Bannigan and Moores, 2009). To illustrate its use in supervision, please see the **Editor's Reflective Story**: Using the Model of Professional Thinking **(Box 6.10)** and **Appendix 6.2** for an accompanying guidance template.

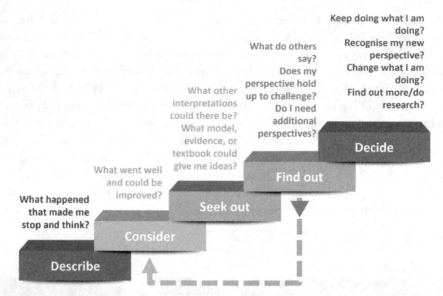

FIGURE 6.3 The Model of Professional Thinking (adapted from Bannigan and Moores, 2009)

BOX 6.10

Editor's Reflective Story: Using the Model of Professional Thinking

In my current role as a university lecturer, I (Karina) often guide students in the classroom and during fieldwork. In this role I am always discussing the importance of reflection and using evidence-based practice. I do find it is easy to say, 'be reflective and use evidence', but acknowledge that it is much harder to do!

I found the Model of Professional Thinking invaluable as I attempted to break down the reflective process and encourage my supervisees (students or practising occupational therapists) to think beyond an inward-looking cycle of 'what did I do well and what could I improve?'. Here is how I explain the key elements of the model, recognising that this all happens within the person's context.

Describe (What?)

Describe an 'event' (experience / incident / conversation / unexpected outcome) that left you with unsettling thoughts or feelings, anxiety, joy, or anger. What happened? Try to stick to the facts and not stray into what you wished might have happened.

Consider (So what?)

Considering what went well and what could be improved is where the analysis of the event begins. We need to pay attention to the feelings that the event brought up for us. In my experience, this inward-looking step, while important, is often where people end their reflection.

Seek out (So what?)

Based on what went well or not so well, seek out (read again) different interpretations from research, theories and/or models. This encourages you to look at the main topic (e.g. communication skills, knowledge of a diagnosis, or intervention technique, etc.) from a wider knowledge base (e.g. from textbooks and/or literature). Does this reading give you a different idea, affirmation of an idea, new thinking, or a different perspective to the situation?

Find out (So what?)

Find out others' opinions on your initial ideas and how this has been informed by your research by discussing with another person such as a supervisor or peer. This sharing is a way for you to sense-check your current understanding of the situation and gain feedback.

In my opinion, this is one of the most valuable steps as it helps people articulate what they are now thinking, and have it affirmed or challenged before considering what to do next. If you have different ideas after your discussions, you may like to return to the 'consider' and 'seek out' steps if you need more information before proceeding.

Decide (Now what?)

After thinking through the situation on your own, seeking out knowledge, and gaining new perspectives from others, the final step is deciding what to do next. It may be that you are doing fine, and this process affirmed what you were doing already, so no need to change. You may have gained a new perspective which changed your existing attitudes or thinking (like the discussion earlier about transformational learning). The process could mean you intend to make a change in your practice, and you could create an action plan to do this. Or you see the need for further learning and/or formal research.

The next section will explore active listening and effective questioning. These are essential skills for the supervisor to develop, although the supervisee may also find some helpful information for developing their own skills for use either in supervision and/or in their professional work.

ACTIVE LISTENING AND EFFECTIVE QUESTIONING

As any relationship is strengthened by clear communication, it is no surprise that clear and effective communication is important during supervision. Asking questions and giving full attention to the supervisee's account of their practice, noticing not only their interpretation, but also the way they are thinking (judgements, assumptions) and feeling (emotional responses) is vital.

Active listening is a core therapeutic skill and something that you will be familiar with. Active listening when a supervisee discloses the challenges faced or debriefs after critical events is a sign that the supervisor cares about their experience. This can impact the level of support the supervisee feels. We have suggested a few ways that could be used to demonstrate active listening in **Box 6.11**. For a more detailed account of active listening and other communication strategies we found the section on communication within *Occupational Performance Coaching: A Manual for Practitioners and Researchers* by Fiona Graham, Ann Kennedy-Behr, and Jenny Ziviani (2020) helpful.

BOX 6.11

Effective listening principles

- Be alert and curious about what the other person is saying.
- Avoid over-sharing your own thoughts, stories, or opinions.
- Focus on the other person: give your complete attention to the speaker.
- Allow the speaker to fully finish before planning your response.
- Pauses and silence are OK and often a useful tool to help the speaker finish their thoughts.

Active listening allows the supervisor to ask well targeted questions. Asking questions helps you to understand the supervisee's perspectives and their reasoning. There are many ways to ask questions and we will provide examples throughout this book to illustrate how you might raise certain topics or explore what is happening within supervision. Frameworks such as coaching and appreciative, strengths-based approaches offer further guidance when it comes to asking questions (please see chapters 2, 7, and 8).

Active listening and effective questioning are important skills of the supervisor in any situation. However, if you are using telesupervision, there may be some additional elements for you to consider. Previous studies, including a systematic review (Martin et al., 2018), have offered some recommendations to enhance communication within telesupervision arrangements, and these are summarised in **Box 6.12**.

BOX 6.12

Techniques for enhancing communication in telesupervision (adapted from Martin et al., 2018)

- Using a clear and slow speaking style.
- Speaking in longer blocks of dialogue.
- Using silence to allow thinking/processing time. It is helpful to discuss how silence may be used and it may take a few sessions to become comfortable with this approach. Try pausing to write notes or taking a sip of water to 'fill the space' if this is more comfortable for you.
- Writing down important comments and decisions or recording the session to capture the discussion for future reference.

- Deliberately taking turns to speak.
- Emailing important information to each other prior to the session.
- Allowing time to become confident and competent in using technology.
- Keeping sessions concise and tackling only a few points at each meeting.

To illustrate the power of active listening and effective questioning in supervision, we invite you to read the **Reflective Story** by an experienced supervisor, Áine O'Dea, as she shares her experience with Tara **(Box 6.13)**.

BOX 6.13

Reflective Story by Áine O'Dea: The power of listening to the supervisee

I was working with an experienced occupational therapist (Tara, a pseudonym) who came to supervision feeling very frustrated and angry. She was working with a family of a child, Ruben (also a pseudonym) with complex needs who had lodged a complaint about her service delivery. I encouraged Tara to tell the story of what had happened leading up to the complaint.

Tara was addressing occupational participation goals relating to mealtimes and going on family outings, and Ruben's seating needs were the priority to support these goals. Tara described a stressful atmosphere during intervention sessions, as communication with the father (Joe, another pseudonym) was difficult. Tara felt that Joe was defensive; he spoke over her and addressed the male equipment representative during the session. Tara felt that Joe often challenged her professional opinion, and it was difficult to identify solutions to the complexity of Ruben's seating needs.

I listened carefully to Tara's story and empathised with the challenges she faced. I acknowledged the complexity of the situation and provided Tara with a safe space to narrate the story. Tara knew when she started working with the family that Joe had made complaints in the past. As Tara reflected on recent sessions, she became increasingly aware of how "what she had done" and "not done" affected each session's outcomes. Tara felt that she had limited the opportunity for Joe to be involved as she had not asked him what piece(s) of equipment he wanted to trial first. She also reflected how she did not make enough effort to develop rapport, citing that she had rarely asked him about his week when he arrived for an appointment. Tara felt that this was an unconscious reaction, as she had anticipated that she would become overwhelmed with "a barrage of unrelated issues" in response to her question.

As I listened, I gathered information and observed Tara's reactions. This information helped me to know how to guide Tara's awareness and reflections of critical points. I used a range of supervision strategies such as prompts, clarifying questions, paraphrasing, and summarising the key points, enabling Tara to identify solutions to address the conflict within the therapeutic relationship. An example included, "I hear you say that you talk more when you are stressed or nervous. I wonder if Joe is also stressed?".

By encouraging a non-judgemental and trusting environment, Tara openly described her experience of the situation. This led to greater awareness about how her values were influencing the case. Tara was able to reframe the interaction and see things from Joe's perspective. Together, we discussed and challenged how some of her underlying assumptions and interpretations had unconsciously swayed her perspective and actions. At the end of the session, we documented Tara's reflections and the solutions she generated (listed below).

Tara's solutions and goals for the subsequent intervention with the family

- Use simple breathing exercises to regulate herself before the start of the next appointment.
- Review her plan for the next appointment and identify how she could allocate 'listening time' for Joe during the session.
- Observe how she listens to Joe during her next session.
- Engage Joe and ask if he valued the sessions, and what changes they could make to the intervention. She planned to acknowledge the complaint and ask if there was anything she could do to help the situation.
- Make written notes of the important points during the session to prevent her from interrupting Joe and offering solutions. Listen to his perceptions and experiences.

Supervision outcomes

Tara reported greater clarity in seeing the family's perspective at the end of the supervision session. Also, she did not feel as angry about the complaint and felt more motivated to try to re-engage with the family.

Active listening and effective questioning are complemented by effective ways to give and receive feedback. In this final skill area, we will explore practical ways to guide learning through feedback.

GIVING AND RECEIVING FEEDBACK

Feedback has historically taken centre stage when it comes to supervision. Feedback has several functions and is an important tool for supervisors to help **bring things into the supervisee's awareness**. It also offers alternatives to current thoughts, ideas, and actions; provides opportunities to modify and change; and supports professional and personal growth (Proctor, 2010). A supervisor is responsible for offering, and being receptive to, feedback.

While feedback is a helpful approach, we need to consider how to make it effective. **Providing a stream of advice and commenting on every action the supervisee is doing is not helpful**. Indeed, some of our thinking around using appreciative, strengths-based or coaching approaches would actively discourage providing this kind of 'advice'. To illustrate the experience of receiving advice in a less than ideal manner, we return to Kyrin and her **Reflective Story** about being an engineer and receiving feedback from healthcare supervisors **(Box 6.14)**.

BOX 6.14

Reflective Story by Kyrin Liong: Supportive feedback that relied on developing the working relationship

When I first began my doctoral journey, my thesis required me to work closely with both engineering and healthcare supervisors. Although my healthcare supervisors seemed gentle and compassionate, I found working in a different discipline difficult. I had spent the first few months scrambling to learn the technical speak that came with their world, just so I could keep up in meetings. Despite my healthcare supervisors' attempts to explain key concepts to me, there just seemed to be a certain disconnect in how we were communicating. What seemed patently obvious to them was hardly apparent to me. Likewise, when I thought certain mechanical concepts were so plain that no explanation was necessary, they were often lost and, at times, seemed to think that this was due to my lack of understanding of the healthcare problem, and not their misconceptions.

What I experienced in the healthcare department was a culture that was a lot less nurturing and a lot more critical than I had experienced in engineering. Feedback on a peer's work was often voiced without much tact, and their treatment of each other seemed consumingly competitive. Expectedly, when I had my first presentation to the healthcare team, it was not a smooth experience. The loud and harsh criticism I received that day perhaps helped to make me a better researcher and presenter in the long term, but in the short term I was quite anxious prior to any public speaking engagement. I was simply not prepared for such a lashing from people I perceived to be part of a team, but I quickly learned that this was tied in with their cultural norms.

In time, my direct healthcare supervisors provided me with constructive feedback and guidance. This support, however, took effort to build. I could sense that my healthcare supervisors did not fully trust in me. Perhaps they had had prior unfavourable experiences working with engineers, or maybe they were having just as hard a time understanding my technical language or my working culture as I was understanding theirs. Whatever the reason, I felt like I was kept at arm's length in the initial phase of our working together. It was only after about a year and a half together, when the project was starting to make true progress, did the relationship begin to take a turn.

I remember the exact meeting as clear as day. I had completed my data collection and, in doing so, had found something surprising and novel in the data. When I presented this to my healthcare supervisors, it was the first time they stopped what they were doing, looked up at me and smiled and said, "I think we really have something here." From that point onwards, any matter that I brought forward for discussion was met with a welcoming demeanour, and my questions were not simply answered but taken forward to see if we could come up with more insightful observations together. I believe that is the point collegial trust was established and we truly began to work together as a team.

Kyrin's account of the feedback she received illustrates how remarks, perhaps made in haste and not meant so harshly, can have a significant impact on the supervisee well beyond the time they were made. When you decide feedback is appropriate for the situation, **Box 6.15** offers characteristics of useful feedback for your consideration.

BOX 6.15

Characteristics of useful feedback (adapted from Edmonstone, 2018)

- **Descriptive rather than evaluative**: Focus feedback on behaviours the supervisee can address in some way, e.g. 'I notice that each time you have felt a therapy session didn't go well, you were having a time-pressured day'.
- **Balanced**: Help to highlight what the supervisee is doing well, e.g. 'You seem to develop good relationships with the people you are working with.' As a separate thought (try to not use 'but' after a positive statement as it can reduce the value of the positive feedback) offer ideas about what might need improvement, e.g. 'Sometimes you are not sure of the most suitable intervention for each person'.
- **Specific and timely, but well considered:** Specific feedback may have more impact if it is provided on the spot within the supervision session, or close to

the event if you are observing a supervisee's practice. However, it is critical that it is not a hastily thought through response but informed by a good understanding of the situation. The supervisor may need to ask clarifying questions or observe the supervisee for longer to pick up the subtext in what they are saying and allow insightful feedback.

Pendleton's Feedback Model (Pendleton et al., 2003) provides supervisors with a framework for giving effective feedback. This model encourages a **dialogue between the feedback provider and the receiver**. It puts the supervisee at the centre of their experience, eliciting their perceptions first before the supervisor offers their view. Thus, it can enhance the supportive climate within the supervision relationship and make the supervisee feel valued. **Figure 6.4** provides an overview of the six steps in the model.

In the Pendleton Feedback Model (Pendleton et al., 2003), the supervisor asks the supervisee to describe what went well **(1)**. This not only facilitates self-reflection but also enables the supervisee to offer their version of their experience **(2)**. Following this step, the supervisor adds what went well from their perspective and asks what could be improved **(3)**, actively listening to the supervisee's response **(4)**. The supervisor recognises what went well, adds their own views, or challenges the supervisee's perspectives if needed **(5)**. Finally, the supervisor asks the supervisee to recap on the important elements of the conversation and create an action plan for incorporating the feedback into practice **(6)**.

In preparation for using the Pendleton Feedback Model, you may want to make a note of areas you wish to highlight and think about how you could phrase aspects that went well and areas for improvement. **Appendix 6.3** is a Pendleton feedback guidance template to help prepare for these conversations.

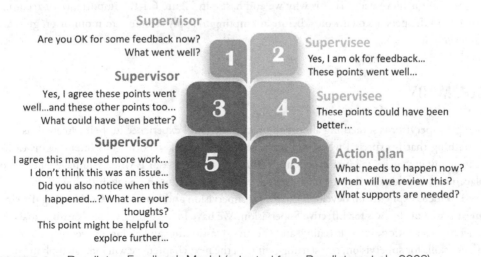

FIGURE 6.4 Pendleton Feedback Model (adapted from Pendleton et al., 2003)

The final section in this chapter is a critical commentary about one of the foundations of occupational therapy practice and a skill we explored at the start of this chapter, goal setting.

CRITICAL COMMENTARY

Are SMART goals a bad idea?

The use of specific parameters to make goals concrete and measurable, such as those represented in the SMART or SMART-ER model are frequently presented as an unarguable practice, yet there are many disadvantages to this method and here are a few reasons why this might be.

Use of the SMART-ER format does not predict someone's success at either a personal or organisational level (Murphy, 2010). Instead, when people in this study were asked, they said that realistic and achievable goals didn't help them achieve great things … they helped them achieve realistic and predictable things that didn't force them out of their comfort zone. SMART-ER goals are generally written with an underlying assumption of achievement. When this is so, achievement often doesn't come with the deep sense of pride or accomplishment.

Humans are not robots, and things seldom conform to the plan that SMART-ER goals presume. True growth also comes from having permission to make decisions, change plans, and experience a healthy dose of daily micro-stresses that lead away from conformity to creativity and problem solving. Indeed, a study by Copley et al. (2021) found that SMART goals with specific measurement increments may not be sensitive enough to capture outcomes that are meaningful for people, and that outcomes need to be evaluated over time. This study was in relation to working with people who access our services, but from our own experiences, we have a feeling that it could be true when applied in our own lives.

While SMART and SMART-ER goals provide a useful framework (and we are not suggesting we abandon this altogether), remember that the intent in goal setting is to promote growth. Having an 'open goal' such as wanting to improve in an area may be more motivating as any progress is seen as an achievement. That is why we emphasise in Figure 6.1 the importance of recording the goal in the person's own words, before attempting to apply structure to monitor progress and achievement.

SUMMARY

Being a supervisor is something almost all practitioners will experience in their careers. It is often something that is expected when you reach a certain level of seniority, but often begins earlier, as in many instances, the first experience you have as a supervisor is when you have students on placement or fieldwork in your organisation. In this chapter, we have taken the position that we need to focus explicitly on developing skills for supervision and hence why **Continuing development** is one of the 3Cs for Effective Supervision. We have focused on creating learning goals and objectives; reflection, active listening, and effective questioning; and giving and receiving feedback as core skills for supervision, as a starting point. In the next chapter, we will look at applying occupational therapy knowledge and skills to enhance supervision by drawing on coaching, creativity, and group work.

REFERENCES

American Occupational Therapy Association (2020) 'Occupational therapy practice framework: domain and process: fourth edition', *American Journal of Occupational Therapy*, 74(2), pp. 7412410010p1–7412410010p87. doi:10.5014/ajot.2020.74S2001.

Atkins, S. and Murphy, K. (1993) 'Reflection: a review of the literature', *Journal of Advanced Nursing*, 18(8), pp. 1188–1192. doi:10.1046/j.1365-2648.1993.18081188.x.

Bannigan, K. and Moores, A. (2009) 'A model of professional thinking: integrating reflective practice and evidence based practice', *Canadian Journal of Occupational Therapy*, 76(5), pp. 342–350. doi:10.1177/000841740907600505.

Bravata, D., Watts, S., Keefer, A.L., Madhusudhan, D.K., Taylor, K., Clark, D., Nelson, R.S., Cokley, K., and Hagg, H.K. (2019) 'Prevalence, predictors, and treatment of impostor syndrome: a systematic review', *Journal of General Internal Medicine*, 35, pp. 1252–1275. doi:10.1007/s11606-019-05364-1.

Carroll, M. (2010a) 'Supervision: critical reflection for transformational learning (part 2)', *The Clinical Supervisor*, 29(1), pp. 1–19. doi:10.1080/07325221003730301.

Carroll, M. (2010b) 'Levels of reflection: on learning reflection', *Psychotherapy in Australia*, 16(2), pp. 24–31. doi:10.3316/informit.727680093884978.

Clance, P.R. and Imes, S.A. (1978) 'The imposter phenomenon in high achieving women: dynamics and therapeutic intervention', *Psychotherapy: Theory, Research & Practice*, 15(3), pp. 241–247. doi:10.1037/h0086006.

Copley, J.A., Nelson, A., Hill, A.E., Castan, C., McLaren, C.F., Brodrick, J., Quinlan, T., and White, R. (2021) 'Reflecting on culturally responsive goal achievement with indigenous clients using the Australian Therapy Outcome Measure for Indigenous Clients (ATOMIC)', *Australian Occupational Therapy Journal*, 68. pp. 384–394. doi:10.1111/1440-1630.12735.

Cox, A. (2005) 'What are communities of practice? A comparative review of four seminal works', *Journal of Information Science*, 31(6), pp. 527–540. doi:10.1177/0165551505057016.

Edmonstone, J. (2018) 'Conferences as sites of learning and development: using participatory action learning and action research approaches', *Action Learning: Research and Practice*, 15(2), pp. 193–197. doi:10.1080/14767333.2018.1464747.

Graham, F., Kennedy-Behr, A., and Ziviani, J. (2020) *Occupational performance coaching: a manual for practitioners and researchers*. Abingdon: Routledge.

Gribble, N. and Netto, J. (2020) 'The preferred method of reflection for occupational therapy students during and after clinical placements: video, written or artistic?', in Billett, S., Orrell, J., Jackson, D., and Valencia-Forrester, F. (eds) *Enriching higher education students' learning through post-work placement interventions*. Cham: Springer, pp. 133–149.

Honey, P. and Mumford, A. (2006) *The learning styles questionnaire: 80-item version*. Maidenhead: Peter Honey.

Husmann, P.R. and O'Loughlin, V.D. (2019) 'Another nail in the coffin for learning styles? Disparities among undergraduate anatomy students' study strategies, class performance, and reported VARK learning styles', *Anatomical Sciences Education*, 12(1), pp. 6–19. doi:10.1002/ase.1777.

Kaelin, V.C. and Dancza, K. (2019) 'Perceptions of occupational therapy threshold concepts by students in role-emerging placements in schools: a qualitative investigation', *Australian Occupational Therapy Journal*, 66, pp. 711–719. doi:10.1111/1440-1630.12610.

Liebel, A.M. (2018) *12 reflective practice prompts for health professionals*. Available at: https://healthcommunicationpartners.com/12-reflective-practice-prompts/ (Accessed: 9 November 2021).

Martin, P., Copley, J., and Tyack, Z. (2014) 'Twelve tips for effective clinical supervision based on a narrative literature review and expert opinion', *Medical Teacher*, 36(3), pp. 201–207. doi:10.3109/0142159X.2013.852166.

Martin, P., Lizarondo, L., and Kumar, S. (2018) 'A systematic review of the factors that influence the quality and effectiveness of telesupervision for health professionals', *Journal of Telemedicine and Telecare*, 24(4), pp. 271–281. doi:10.1177/1357633X17698868.

Moon, J. (1999) *Reflection in learning and professional development*. London: Kogan Page.

Moon, J. (2004) *A handbook of reflective and experiential learning*. Abingdon: Routledge Falmer.

Moran, M. and Dancza, K. (2018) 'Establishing, finalising or redefining client-centred and occupation-focused goals', in Dancza, K. and Roger, S. (eds) *Implementing occupation-centred practice: a practical guide of occupational therapy practice learning*. London: Routledge, pp. 169–183.

Murphy, M. (2010) *Hard goals: the secret to getting from where you are to where you want to be*. London: McGraw-Hill.

Nicola-Richmond, K., Pépin, G., Larkin, H., and Mohebbi, M. (2019) 'Threshold concept acquisition in occupational therapy: a mixed methods study of students and clinicians', *Australian Occupational Therapy Journal*, 66, pp. 568–580. doi:10.1111/1440-1630.12595.

Pashler, H., McDaniel, M., Rohrer, D., and Bjork, R. (2008) 'Learning styles: concepts and evidence', *Psychological Science in the Public Interest*, 9(3), pp. 105–119. doi:10.1111/j.1539-6053.2009.01038.x.

Pendleton, D., Schofield, T., Tate, P., and Havelock, P. (2003) *The new consultation: developing doctor–patient communication*. Oxford: Oxford University Press.

Proctor, B. (2010) 'Training for the supervision alliance: attitude, skills and intention', in Cutcliffe, J.R., Hyrkas, K., and Fowler, J. (eds) *Routledge handbook of clinical supervision: fundamental international themes*. London: Routledge, pp. 51–62.

Rodger, S., Turpin, M., and O'Brien, M. (2015) 'Experiences of academic staff in using threshold concepts within a reformed curriculum', *Studies in Higher Education*, 40(4), pp. 545–560. doi:10.1080/0307507 9.2013.830832.

Rothwell, C., Kehoe, A., Farook, S. and Illing, J. (2019) *The characteristics of effective clinical and peer supervision in the workplace: a rapid evidence review*. Newcastle: Newcastle University.

Appendix 6.1: Creating learning goals and objectives guidance template

GOAL (IN SUPERVISEE'S OWN WORDS)	
For example: *I want to improve my assessment skills.*	
LEARNING OBJECTIVE (WHAT THE SUPERVISEE WILL DO DIFFERENTLY)	
For example: *Nhungi will demonstrate competency with the administration of the occupational performance analysis tool within 4 weeks.*	
TARGETS (ELEMENTS THAT NEED TO BE DONE TO MEET THE LEARNING OBJECTIVE)	
What steps will be done	Progress review date, outcome, and next steps
For example: *Independently administer the assessment at least twice a week for four weeks; interpret the results of the assessment with minimal prompts; document the results of the assessment with 100% accuracy.*	
SUPPORTIVE ACTIONS	
What will help meet the targets	Who is responsible
For example: *Supervisor will identify opportunities for Nhungi to observe other therapists conducting an occupational performance analysis; time will be set aside during supervision to discuss assessment interpretations; Nhungi will document at least eight assessments, and her supervisor will verify results and check for recording accuracy.*	
PROGRESS REVIEW AND UPDATES	

Appendix 6.2: Model of professional thinking guidance template

1. DESCRIBE	
What happened that made you stop and think? • An event? • Conversation? • Idea?	**Notes:**
2. CONSIDER	
What went well and could be improved? • Your actions? • Your response? • Your thinking? How did the event make you feel?	**Notes:**
3. SEEK OUT	
What other interpretations can you find to understand what happened? • From research, theories and/or models? • Contextual influences? How do these perspectives reinforce, add to, or change your thinking?	**Notes:**
4. FIND OUT	
What do others say about what happened and your current interpretations? • A supervisor? • A peer? • Another professional? Does your perspective hold up to challenge? Do you need additional perspectives from people or literature (go back to consider and seek out)?	**Notes:**
5. DECIDE	
What will you do now? • Keep doing what you are doing • Recognise your new perspective • Change what you are doing • Think about/find out more from new sources • Do formal investigation/research	**Notes:**

Appendix 6.3: Pendleton feedback guidance template

1. SUPERVISOR – ASKS WHAT WENT WELL	
• Are you OK for some feedback now? • What went well?	**Notes:**
2. SUPERVISEE – EXPRESSES WHAT WENT WELL	
• Note supervisee sharing	**Notes:**
3. SUPERVISOR – RESPONDS TO WHAT WENT WELL AND ASKS WHAT COULD BE BETTER	

• Yes, I agree these points went well …
  [review statements made by supervisee
  about what went well]
• I thought these areas were also positive …
  [note before your feedback session]
• Example statements could be:
  o You approached the person and
     made them feel comfortable.
  o Your documentation was clear and
     highlights relevant points.
  o You responded appropriately in that
     situation.
  o Your evaluation and
     recommendations are relevant.
  o It was a challenging day, thank you
     for your support.
• What could have been better?
	Notes:

4. SUPERVISEE – EXPRESSES WHAT COULD HAVE BEEN BETTER	
• Note supervisee sharing	**Notes:**
5. SUPERVISOR – RESPONDS TO WHAT COULD BE BETTER AND ASKS WHAT NEXT	

• Yes, I agree this may need more work …
  [review supervisee statements]
• I don't think these points were an issue …
  [challenge any points you felt were OK]
• Did you notice when … [highlight an
  important issue that hasn't been raised]
  happened? What do you think about it?
• I also thought … [this point] would be
  useful to discuss further
• Example statements could be:
  o It is important to introduce your role
     clearly but briefly.
  o Try to focus on one point at a time.
  o We can discuss ways of coping when
     you feel overwhelmed.
  o Let's work through a report and see
     how it can flow better.
• What needs to happen now? When will
  we review this?
• What support do you need from me?
	Notes:

6. SUPERVISEE – SHARES THEIR ACTION PLAN	
• Note supervisee sharing of action plan	**Notes:**

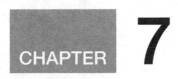

CHAPTER 7

Applying occupational therapy knowledge and skills to enhance supervision

Karina Dancza, Sarah Harvey, Áine O'Dea, Anita Volkert, and Merrolee Penman

With contributions from Ann Kennedy-Behr

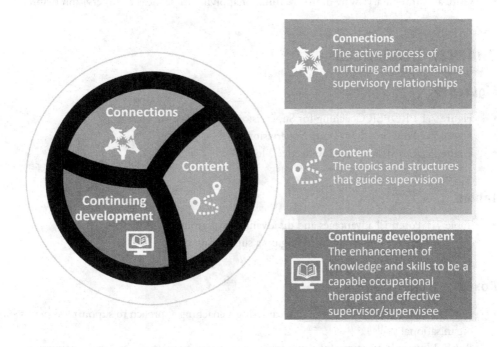

Connections
The active process of nurturing and maintaining supervisory relationships

Content
The topics and structures that guide supervision

Continuing development
The enhancement of knowledge and skills to be a capable occupational therapist and effective supervisor/supervisee

DOI: 10.4324/9781003092544-7

CHAPTER INTENTIONS

In this chapter, we invite you to:

- Reflect on your occupational therapy knowledge and skills and how they can be applied to enhance supervision
- Review coaching, creative, and group approaches, and consider their potential use in supervision
- Explore ways to explicitly introduce and embed different ways of doing supervision in practice.

CHAPTER HIGHLIGHTS

- Supervision using what we already know and do
- Coaching approaches in supervision
- Creative approaches in supervision
- Group approaches in supervision
- Critical commentary: Why didn't we think of applying these ideas to supervision before?

CHAPTER RESOURCES

Figures

- Figure 7.1 PROPER Coaching for Supervision Framework
- Figure 7.2 Four Steps for Group Supervision
- Figure 7.3 Discussion-Based Reflective Model

Tables

- Table 7.1 Potential advantages and disadvantages of groups
- Table 7.2 Where to start when setting up a supervision group

Boxes

- Box 7.1 Reflective Story by Áine O'Dea: Using a coaching approach to support a supervisee's organisational skills
- Box 7.2 Example questions for a supervisee to ask a supervisor/peer during a coaching session
- Box 7.3 Reflective Story by Áine O'Dea: Using a coaching approach from a supervisor's perspective
- Box 7.4 Reflective Story by Ann Kennedy-Behr: Using playfulness in supervision

- Box 7.5 Tips for setting up and conducting role play in supervision
- Box 7.6 Reflective Story by Sarah Harvey: Using groups in multi-professional supervision
- Box 7.7 Example ground rules in group supervision
- Box 7.8 Reflective Story by Sarah Harvey: Processing feelings in group supervision
- Box 7.9 Reflective activities to help prepare for the role of group supervisor

Appendices

- Appendix 7.1 PROPER Coaching for Supervision guidance template
- Appendix 7.2 PROPER Coaching for Supervision documentation template
- Appendix 7.3 Four Steps for Group Supervision guidance template
- Appendix 7.4 Group reflection guidance template

SUPERVISION USING WHAT WE ALREADY KNOW AND DO

As occupational therapists, we draw from a broad knowledge base that covers physical and mental health, lifespan development, science, philosophy, and the arts, to name a few. We also devote a great deal of our energy to the relationships we have with others, as it is by working together that we can create, change, and evolve. With such a broad range of knowledge and skills in working with people, we have so many options when it comes to supervision.

In this chapter, we will be reviewing some common therapeutic tools we use with people who access occupational therapy services and consider how we can apply them in supervision. Specifically, we will be exploring coaching, creative, and group approaches. The intention here is to acknowledge our existing knowledge and skills and make them work for us in supervision.

COACHING APPROACHES IN SUPERVISION

We begin by describing what a coaching approach may look like when used by an occupational therapist in supervision. The idea here is to apply coaching techniques within a supervisory framework (such as the 3Cs for Effective Supervision), rather than acting as a 'coach' for the supervisee. In some situations, it may be preferable for a supervisee to seek out a coach if there are specific areas they wish to work on outside of supervision. We also acknowledge that coaching is a separate discipline (as discussed in Chapter 1). Therefore, we suggest using approaches associated with coaching through the lens of occupational therapy and supervisory practices, unless you decide to formally extend your role with additional coaching credentials.

As a starting point, we invite you to read the **Reflective Story** by Áine O'Dea as she describes her experience as a supervisor using a coaching approach with Maebh (a pseudonym) as she struggles with organising her workload **(Box 7.1)**.

Reflective Story by Áine O'Dea: Using a coaching approach to support a supervisee's organisational skills

Maebh contacted me to provide supervision that was external to her service setting. At the outset, Maebh acknowledged that she had not engaged in supervision in her previous role due to numerous organisational barriers. Maebh was nervous and unsure if she was up to date with evidence-based knowledge, and she wanted to address this in supervision.

During the first couple of sessions, Maebh struggled to prepare an agenda before supervision, reporting that she was too busy. Maebh spoke about numerous aspects of her work in a disorganised and brief manner, quickly jumping from one topic to another.

As a supervisor, I focused my attention on listening to Maebh's narratives. As Maebh spoke, I realised that she found it difficult to reflect on her practice. She described numerous case scenarios, detailing what happened, what she did, and what others did. Moving to the next stage of reflection, which involved analysing and making sense of her observations and feelings about the case scenario, proved more difficult.

During our initial sessions, I observed and acknowledged to Maebh that she knew a lot of factual details about her caseload. However, it seemed like she was a little overwhelmed. I noted that Maebh had an incredible memory, which was her predominant means of organising her daily and weekly interactions. I was also curious to know if she received any support to help manage her workload.

At this stage in supervision, I was conscious of gaining Maebh's trust (**Connection**) before moving on to using a coaching approach (**Content**) to help her move forward. I empathised with the hectic nature of her work and limited resources. I gently encouraged Maebh to consider what it was like to manage such a busy workload. I did not offer solutions or tell her what to do as I recognised that it would potentially reinforce Maebh's insecurity and increase her stress.

Instead, I asked Maebh carefully chosen open questions to find out if she had any ideas about how she could reduce the busyness of her day. Her response was that she was unsure of what she could do to improve things. Taking things at a pace Maebh was OK with, we agreed that she would consciously observe her workload, the number of interactions that occurred per day, etc., until our next supervision session.

As our relationship developed and Maebh gained trust that I was not going to judge her or tell her what she should do and, we were able to make some useful progress. Introducing a coaching style to the structure of supervision enabled Maebh to think of and start using some organisational strategies to support her caseload management and reduce work-related stress. Over time this progress enhanced her confidence and productivity as an occupational therapist (**Continuing development**).

Coaching has attracted attention in occupational therapy in recent years as a strategy for working with people in health and social care contexts (Graham et al., 2020). There are many forms of coaching available, including Occupational Performance Coaching, which was developed within occupational therapy. In this approach, the focus is on working towards goals through amplifying the expertise and agency of the person to select what is important, analyse the situation, make decisions about what to change, and monitor the success of those actions (Graham et al., 2020). Other coaching approaches have been developed outside of occupational therapy, such as the GROW model (Grant, 2011; Whitmore, 1992), Early Childhood Coaching (Rush and Shelden, 2011), Solution-Focused Coaching in Pediatric Rehabilitation (King et al., 2019), and many others. You may be familiar with some coaching principles even if you do not specially use one approach.

As there are many ways to undertake a coaching conversation in supervision, we propose our own summary of the key steps in the **PROPER Coaching for Supervision [Priority, Reality, Opportunities, Plan, Evaluate, Review]** Framework (**Figure 7.1**). The PROPER Coaching for Supervision Framework is a six-step approach where the supervisor and supervisee work in partnership to: (**1**) identify a **priority** topic, (**2**) explore the **reality** of what is happening now, (**3**) consider **opportunities** for making a change, (**4**) create a **plan** of action, (**5**) **evaluate** confidence and competence for doing the plan, and (**6**) **review** progress in follow-up sessions.

This original diagram (Figure 7.1) drew much of its inspiration from the GROW model (Whitmore, 1992) and Occupational Performance Coaching (Graham et al., 2020). The diagram offers a few prompts to guide the conversation, and **Appendix 7.1** presents additional questions in the form of a **PROPER Coaching for Supervision guidance template**. We have also suggested a record-keeping format in **Appendix 7.2**: PROPER Coaching for Supervision documentation template.

A critical element of coaching is **trying not to problem-solve for the person or present your own solutions**; rather guiding the person to come to their own ideas and answers. The importance of this point can be highlighted if you think back to a time where you have received some unwanted advice from a supervisor, family member, colleague, or friend. When you talk an issue through with someone, often you do not need them to solve the problem for you, you just want them to listen as you talk and perhaps ask a few well-considered questions that prompt you to think about the issue from another perspective. You are more likely to make a change when you have come up with the ideas and solutions.

Coaching approaches can be useful in a one-to-one supervisory session or could be used in combination with group supervision which we will discuss later in this chapter. Now we will consider what coaching feels like from the perspectives of the supervisee and supervisor.

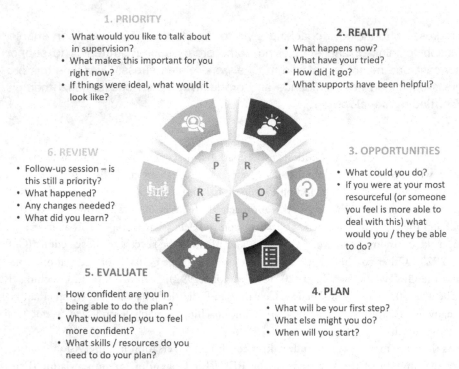

FIGURE 7.1 PROPER Coaching for Supervision Framework (developed from Whitmore, 1992; Graham et al., 2020)

Coaching from the supervisee perspective

Being coached may feel different from other forms of supervision. It is anticipated that, as a supervisee being coached, you will be doing a lot of the talking and thinking. Your supervisor may not offer as much advice or as many ideas as perhaps you are used to in another version of supervision. You will be encouraged to think about what is important to you, reflect on the realities of what is happening, and think of things that you could do to make a change. The major benefit of this approach for the supervisee is that you draw from your own knowledge and strengths while still considering other perspectives to guide or reframe your thinking. This can be a very empowering experience, as you create your own understandings of the situation or experience.

Even though you are encouraged to think about your own situation and potential, it does not mean that you need to ignore or avoid the opinions of your supervisor, or peers and colleagues if you are in a group supervision situation. **You can ask questions** (see examples in **Box 7.2**) to help you see the situation from different perspectives and think through alternative solutions.

BOX 7.2

Example questions for a supervisee to ask a supervisor/peer during a coaching session

- What do you think my next step might be?
- What do you think might be the likely outcome of this?
- Who might help me to get there?
- What strengths do you think I can draw from?
- What have others done in a similar situation?
- What do you think is stopping me getting there?
- What theory or literature do you think could offer me new insights?

Coaching from the supervisor perspective

Intentionally using a coaching approach can mean a change in how we 'do' supervision. As a supervisor, we may have gravitated towards sharing our skills and knowledge with a less experienced supervisee. The temptation to tell a supervisee what to do can be hard to resist. However, it changes the power dynamic in the supervisory relationship.

As a supervisor, you can ask the supervisee questions that bring ideas to their awareness. This careful questioning and strategic sharing of perspectives or information provides the supervisee with a graded approach to evaluating their practice and is the precursor to significant learning and professional development. When the supervisory relationship is open and non-judgemental we can encourage supervisees to work towards their goals through magnifying their expertise and agency to select what is important, analyse the situation, make decisions about what to change, and monitor the success of those actions. We return to another **Reflective Story** by Áine O'Dea as she describes her view of using a coaching approach as a supervisor (**Box 7.3**).

BOX 7.3

Reflective Story by Áine O'Dea: Using a coaching approach from a supervisor's perspective

A critical learning and development point occurred when I read about Occupational Performance Coaching within Sylvia Rodger's book *Occupation-Centred Practice with Children* (Rodger, 2010; Graham et al., 2010). Graham describes the importance of mindful listening, non-judgemental acceptance, and authentic expression of empathy to support relationship development with the client (Graham et al., 2020). The parallel within the supervision process was striking. Reflecting upon my practice as a supervisor, I noted that in the early stages of working with a new supervisee, numerous sessions could be required to establish trust in the supervisory relationship, as I described in my account of supervising Maebh.

Once this relationship was established, using a coaching approach I was opening opportunities for Maebh to discover her own solutions and ways of doing things (i.e. ask, don't tell). My expertise shifted from knowing what the supervisee needed to develop, to knowing how to engage the supervisee to determine what is important and how to make changes to their own situation (Graham, 2020). While at times I wanted to give lots of advice, the more familiar I became with coaching the more comfortable I was to guide and create space for the supervisee to find their own way.

In our next section, looking at applying our occupational therapy knowledge and skills in supervision we will be focusing on using creative approaches to bring different perspectives to supervisory sessions.

CREATIVE APPROACHES IN SUPERVISION

Creativity in supervision leads to new insights, meanings, ideas, and courses of action beyond what happens with traditional approaches (Scaife, 2019). Creativity can come in the form of talking in different ways or using other materials as guides and prompts for challenging thinking, visualising things differently, and critically analysing existing practices. Creativity can be particularly helpful if a supervisee is 'stuck' in a situation or perspective, or if the supervisor wants to enhance what they can offer and prevent themselves from becoming stale. As an introduction to using creativity in supervision, we invite you to read the **Reflective Story** by Ann Kennedy-Behr as she describes how she uses creativity and playfulness as a tool in her supervisory practices **(Box 7.4)**.

BOX 7.4

Reflective Story by Ann Kennedy-Behr: Using playfulness in supervision

I wished I had been more playful as a supervisor. I felt the responsibility weighed heavily on me and that did not translate well in my interactions with supervisees. As a therapist, I consciously used playfulness as a therapeutic tool. I have always managed this playfulness when in a therapy role (I have worked primarily as an occupational therapist with children) but found it more challenging in a supervisory role. I had a fear of my supervisees not taking the work seriously or pushing boundaries, especially when working with groups such as occupational therapy students.

Playfulness to me means approaching things creatively, taking a light-hearted approach, playing with words and ideas. I found that this style relaxed people, made them feel we were on the same team, gave them opportunities to laugh in otherwise bleak moments, and kept them engaged. There was always a risk that a light-hearted approach may offend some, but that rarely happened; the key seemed to be in acknowledging serious situations while still maintaining a sense of the ridiculousness that life sometimes throws at us.

A mentor once suggested that I view my supervisees as people with therapeutic goals. This reframing was in itself a playful approach – considering a situation from an unexpected point of view. On reflection, I could have used games to create group identity and strengthen relationships, particularly between those supervisees who didn't know each other well. I could have looked at incorporating playful elements into tasks, deliberately imposing constraints to make a challenge ('construct an assistive device using just three household items'; write ten SMART goals in ten minutes!) or more importantly, encourage the supervisee to see the pleasure in the problem-solving that is so inherent in the occupational therapy process.

Creative and playful supervision does not have to mean the use of specific techniques. It can simply be in the perspectives taken; holding the weight of responsibility lightly; taking the role, but not oneself, seriously; and remembering that supervisees, just like the people who access our services, need to feel they are on the same team, need opportunities to laugh. Using creative and playful strategies may help supervisees move beyond description and towards reflection on what happened and making sense of it from different perspectives. Our starting point for creative ideas is something that we are perhaps already quite familiar with – reflective writing.

Reflective writing

The use of reflective writing is common when working with occupational therapy students. However, it may also be something that was completed as a requirement, rather than seen as a useful learning strategy. It may be helpful to revisit reflective writing in a way that offers choice and freedom for the supervisee. Templates of reflective questions can offer structure for the supervisee and supervisor (as discussed in Chapter 6). Reflective writing can also be facilitated in a group situation using techniques such as setting out large pieces of paper or whiteboards around the room. You can ask people to write or draw ideas, thoughts, feelings, key learning points, or anything else about the topic on the wall. The supervisor can then facilitate discussions based on what is presented. Reflections do not always have to be completed with words. Beyond writing, illustrations, and diagrams (without comment on artistic flair!), along with an opportunity to debrief, can add some variety to supervision activities.

Visual representations

Sometimes supervisees may experience challenges putting their experiences into words. One strategy is to **create a diagram, drawing, mind map, or other visual representation** of the scenario or situation. Seeing the information in a different way has the potential to help someone consider issues or opportunities for success and change from multiple perspectives. Discussions based on these visual representations could explore what is known about the scenario or situation by asking the supervisee to share or explain elements of the image or what happened before or after the snapshot presented, as well as what connections between different elements emerge as part of the discussions.

In occupational therapy, we use a range of visual tools when exploring the occupational lives of the people who access our services. For example, some have used the **KAWA model** (Iwama et al., 2009) and its river metaphor to explore a situation with a person. Using supervision time to co-create the metaphor or asking the supervisee to prepare something in advance are both helpful. Supervisees – either individually or as a group – contribute significant events, positive or negative influences, or other characteristics that have shaped the journey by adding text or drawings to the river. After the initial draft, debriefing is important, and this can happen with the supervisor or during peer or group supervision. **Visual representations can be altered** based on this discussion and any new insights achieved.

Visual representations may also include **tangible objects**. Experimenting with the use of clay, sand, magnets on a board, or even figurines could introduce a playful element to supervision. You may like to start with something familiar, such as making the KAWA river in clay. The supervisee can create, use, and arrange the objects to help explain a work situation or relationship that they wish to discuss. The supervisor could ask questions about the arrangement such as, 'What would happen if this object moved somewhere else?' or 'What would happen if this person was bigger/ smaller?'. The aim is to see situations from different perspectives and identify potential elements for change (Scaife, 2019).

Role play

Role play is another potentially creative addition to supervision. Role plays are where people enact or rehearse a practical component of their work from either the perspective of the therapist or person accessing the service (Bearman et al., 2013). Role play may also include watching others demonstrate a strategy (Bennett-Levy et al., 2009).

Role plays of therapeutic scenarios can be guided through three stages, **(1) building rapport**, where the conversation is general, **(2) critical conversation/event**, where the focus of therapy is practised, and **(3) sharing**, where all parties debrief about the scenario. **Box 7.5** offers tips for setting up and conducting a role play activity in supervision.

> ### BOX 7.5
>
> ### Tips for setting up and conducting role play in supervision (adapted from Andersson et al., 2010)
>
> - The role play scenario can be mutually agreed, based on the learning needs of the supervisee(s).
> - Turn taking between being the therapist and person receiving the service can be a helpful strategy to enable people to see things from both perspectives.
> - Working in a group of three – therapist, person receiving service, and observer – can be effective. The observer can lead the sharing and offer insights that may be different from the main players.
> - Using a feedback structure such as Pendleton's Model (see Chapter 6) can be an effective way to structure the sharing stage of role play.

Teaching others is another useful learning strategy that can be included in a role play. For example, a supervisee may teach a peer or supervisor about a therapy technique they are trying to master. The act of explaining it to someone else often helps to clarify and consolidate their own understanding.

Evidence on the use of active strategies such as role play in supervision and other educational activities is promising. For example, Bearman et al. (2013) reported on a study investigating the use of role play and expert modelling in supervision and found that these strategies increased the likelihood that practices will be done in sessions as planned. Milne et al. (2011) also suggested that educational role play and modelling were helpful methods for use in supervision. Creative approaches can also work well in group supervision situations, and this is the final area we will explore.

GROUP APPROACHES IN SUPERVISION

Group supervision can offer opportunities for peer support and sharing a range of perspectives. It may also be viewed as a cost-effective method of offering supervision. Group supervision can comprise a combination of participants, such as a group of peers, colleagues with a range of experience levels, an interprofessional team, or multiple supervisors to multiple supervisees. A variety of approaches is also possible such as using action learning sets (Haith and Whittingham, 2012, see Chapter 5), communities of practice (Cox, 2005, see Chapter 6), or Balint groups (Salinsky, 2009). In this section we will draw on our skills in group facilitation and apply them in a supervision scenario. While not necessarily a new idea, we hope that this section offers a useful reminder, or a starting point, to try out ideas in your own context.

You may already be familiar with one of the most influential theories of group processes proposed by Tuckman (1965). This was originally a four-stage sequential model, (latterly a five-stage model – see Tuckman and Jensen, 1977) which outlines the common tasks and social behaviours of a group:

1. **Forming** – Where people become orientated to the group and get to know each other. There are uncertainties and people look for direction and leadership, while considering what they might be expected to do and what they can gain from the group.
2. **Storming** – This can be a difficult stage to navigate as it is where people may disagree on group goals, subgroups form and individual personalities are shown. Group productivity may decrease during this phase. It is important to address conflict and competition for the group to move forward.
3. **Norming** – The group comes together and resolves enough of the storming conflicts to form a functioning group structure (e.g. leaders, individual roles). Cooperation and a focus on the group goals emerge, although tensions may still arise and push the group back into the storming stage.
4. **Performing** – Consensus and collaboration are well established, and the group is functioning well. The group is working productively and tensions, when they arise, are handled constructively.
5. **Adjourning** – Most of the group goals are achieved and the group is preparing to finish their work together. Acknowledgement of successes and contributions often marks the end of the group. If the group is ongoing but the membership changes, then the group may enter the forming stage again (Donald and Carter, 2020).

In group supervision, Tuckman and Jensen's (1977) group stages can help us understand how the group is evolving and what is needed from a supervisor during this process. In our first **Reflective Story** of this section, we hear from Sarah Harvey about her experiences of supervision in a multi-professional group, when the group is largely in the 'performing stage' (**Box 7.6**).

BOX 7.6

Reflective Story by Sarah Harvey: Using groups in multi-professional supervision

As an occupational therapist working in acute and community mental health settings, I have experienced group supervision a few times in my career, both as supervisor and supervisee. One example of being a supervisee was working in a mental health setting with a multi-professional team, including occupational therapists, occupational therapy instructors/assistants, nurses, psychologists, and art therapists. The team was working with the same people accessing services, so it made sense for us to share our insights in group supervision discussions.

These group discussions were extremely helpful when we had a situation when someone found a group member hiding sharp objects, taken from the occupational therapy session, with the intention to self-harm. Or when a young man with a mental health diagnosis was communicating inappropriately with young female health professionals in the team. In team meetings, we would discuss the risks and manage them accordingly; however, the group supervision was a place to discuss the feelings we experienced when working with people in distress: our worries about personal safety and the embarrassment of experiencing inappropriate attention. These discussions allowed us to formulate intervention strategies together and re-establish therapeutic boundaries.

The supervisor was a psychologist whose role was to maintain the group's boundaries, make sure we ran to time, and ensure turn taking was observed. The supervisor also helped the group to feel safe to share personal experiences in relation to the people we were working with. They encouraged us to explore any feelings of frustration or sadness and helped us to consider where they came from and how they impacted our work.

What was interesting, yet challenging at the same time, was the different perspectives people brought to supervision. This required careful handling by the supervisor as they facilitated discussions about our knowledge, strengths, and gaps. They helped us explore times when our interventions or communications were successful or had failed. What was reinforced to me was how I was confident in some aspects of my practice (e.g. occupational engagement); however, I had much less confidence in other areas (e.g. risk management). It turned out that other professionals had similar experiences of feeling confident in some areas and not others, and it was only through these supervision conversations were we able to draw from each other strengths to improve our responses to the complex situations we often faced.

Advantages and disadvantages of groups

Group supervision can be beneficial for the diversity of perspectives it encourages, as Sarah outlined in her story. In other situations, it may be that group supervision is the only possible option, because access to supervisors is limited. It is important to consider the potential advantages and disadvantages of group supervision (initial ideas are suggested in **Table 7.1**), so that you can make an informed decision about committing time to this format.

Setting up a supervision group

Critical to the success of the group is how it is planned. Group membership and engagement are supported **when the group is accessible, reliable, and offers a consistent and accommodating environment**. Trying to bring together a group of busy practitioners is no easy feat; therefore, you may need to do some provisional consultation on availability and decide on a physical or virtual space. **Table 7.2** offers additional thoughts about where to start.

How to run a group supervision session

When setting up group supervision, we can apply our knowledge, skills, and frameworks of running groups as a guide. For example, Cole (2017) suggested seven steps when running an occupational therapy group. Inspired by these steps, we propose **Four Steps for Group Supervision** (**Figure 7.2**). These steps are intended as a guide (rather than strict rules) to conducting a session.

TABLE 7.1 Potential advantages and disadvantages of groups

Potential advantages of groups	Potential disadvantages of groups
There are opportunities to explore a range of different perspectives and people can learn from each other in a social atmosphere.	Confidentiality is harder to maintain as there are more people hearing the discussions.
Offers a sense of community, i.e. 'I am not the only one who is experiencing this'.	People may feel less comfortable to share in a group.
Gain feedback, support, challenge, and motivation for change.	It is harder to build trust and safety to share personal perspectives and professional challenges.
Cost- / time-effectiveness.	Time may be insufficient to deal with each person's needs thoroughly, and finding a time when all people are available could be problematic.
People can come together and work on a common issue.	Risks that people will experience peer pressure to conform to the group's view.
The supervisor(s) may benefit from the support of the group in carrying out their role.	Not all people will get along with each other.

TABLE 7.2 Where to start when setting up a supervision group

When will it run?	Busy teams and established workloads are difficult to negotiate. Consistency in scheduling can help it become a routine commitment. Management support and protected time also demonstrate the value of supervision and can impact on people's availability.
Frequency?	A useful question to ask first is, 'How often will the group need this supervision?'. Monthly sessions will ensure consistency for a closed group. If the group is running as an open rolling group for people to dip in and out of, then you may consider a more frequent option.
Group number?	There is no magic number, but if the group is drawn from a large multidisciplinary team, you may wish to consider a larger open group, so more people have the potential to attend. If this group is for a small team, then a smaller closed group membership may be more appropriate.
How long will the sessions be?	There is no set timeframe for group supervision. Group size may dictate the time needed for people to feel like they have been able to adequately contribute. Online sessions may need to be shorter to maintain people's attention. As a rough guide, you may like to start with between 45–90-minute sessions and monitor how effective it is, adjusting the time as needed.

They are: **(1) welcome, (2) main activity, (3) exploration, (4) application and next steps** (see **Appendix 7.3** for a Four Steps for Group Supervision guidance template). In our discussions we will assume that there is one supervisor to a group of supervisees. However, it is also possible to share the supervisor role and co-facilitate sessions as this could present a useful opportunity for professional development of the supervisor.

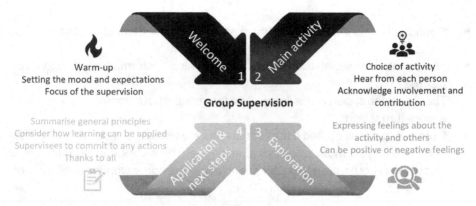

FIGURE 7.2 Four Steps for Group Supervision (adapted from Cole, 2017)

Welcome

Warm-up

The warm-up will depend on how well participants know each other and how much they have previously bonded as a group. Welcoming people, ensuring everyone knows each other's names and maybe something about themselves helps to acknowledge membership in the group and invites everyone to contribute. A **warm-up exercise** can help capture the group's attention, help people relax, and prepare for more serious discussions to follow. Warm-up activities could be general conversations, or you might use creative activities or short games to help create an atmosphere of spontaneity and fun. In subsequent meetings, a recap of previous sessions could also be a useful warm-up for the group (Cole, 2017).

Setting the mood and expectations

Paying attention to the environment is important (e.g. lighting, temperature, noise, privacy, layout of the room, clutter, etc.). If the group supervision is online, you may like to orientate supervisees to their own environment to help them settle before discussions begin (Cole, 2017). When setting the mood and expectations, **ground rules** can be helpful (Cole, 2017). Some topics you may like to raise are included in **Box 7.7**.

BOX 7.7

Example ground rules in group supervision

- Discussions will be appreciative and strengths-based, where problems and challenges are acknowledged, but the focus will be on the strengths of people.
- Everyone is free to share, and different perspectives are valued.

- Confidentiality is important and there should be agreement about this with the group.
- The intention of supervision is not primarily about information provision, but discussion and sharing.
- The role of the supervisor is to maintain the group's boundaries, time keep, and ensure turn taking.
- Online etiquette is agreed if appropriate, such as raising hands, using the chat feature, being on mute when not speaking, etc. It is important to have some discussion about maintaining confidentiality in the home working environment.

Focus of the group

Determining what topics will be covered in the group supervision together with all participants is ideal so that the needs of the group can be addressed. However, in the early stages, the focus could also be something a supervisor introduces in advance of the meeting, so people have time to think and prepare. Topics could include **skill areas, a project or service, cases, situations, theory, a new approach, a research paper, a guideline, etc**. During the session, the group can also review what outcomes people hope to achieve, such as new ideas, sharing achievements, planning a way forward, etc. **Peer pressure** can be a powerful motivator (Cole, 2017) and the group can support each other to commit to, monitor, and achieve their supervision goals.

Main activity

Planning the main activity so that it takes around half of the time you have for the session will mean you have time for the welcome, exploration, and application steps (Cole, 2017). Therefore, for bigger topics you may wish to plan more than one session.

The choice of activity is often influenced by the experience and comfort of the supervisor(s) to lead the session. The group size, topic area, and participant characteristics will also influence how the session proceeds. Supervisees can also take responsibility for leading the activity. There are so many activities that you could try, and a few ideas were presented in the previous section on using creativity in supervision. Rather than presenting a long list of ideas, we thought we would focus on something we feel is extremely valuable in supervision, **reflection**. The extension that we offer here is our view on how to apply the reflective process when working in a group.

When thinking about how to facilitate a reflective supervisory discussion in a group, we developed the **Discussion-Based Reflective Model** (**Figure 7.3**). Inspired by the Model of Professional Thinking (Bannigan and Moores, 2009), this model presents a way for people to think and talk through a situation (e.g. incident with a colleague) or set of skills (e.g. supervision or management skills) to make sense of it and learn something for the future.

The key features of the Discussion-Based Reflective Model are to move through steps in a reflective cycle by **(1) describing the situation or skill, (2) seeking different perspectives, (3) making sense of the learning, (4) planning for action, and (5) documenting the learning**.

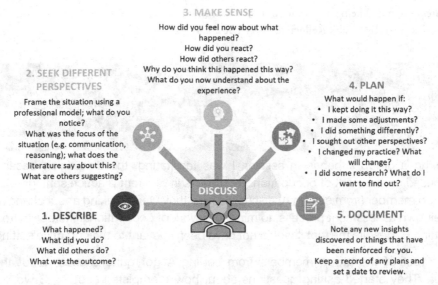

FIGURE 7.3 Discussion-Based Reflective Model (adapted from Bannigan and Moores, 2009)

By placing **discussion** as the central pivot point, we emphasise the importance of social learning (Bandura, 1977), as each element is discussed and debated with peers, colleagues, and/or supervisors. **Appendix 7.4** offers a group reflection guidance template to support you in this activity.

When the main activity is finished, each person is invited to share what they have done (e.g. if the activity was to draw, write, or create something), or summarise what the experience was like for them or meant to them (Cole, 2017). The purpose of sharing is to hear from all supervisees and **acknowledge everyone's involvement and contribution**, although it is OK if people prefer not to share. It is also helpful for the supervisor to hear what the main take-aways were for each person to use in the next step of exploration where any feelings associated with the activity are considered.

Exploration

Exploration involves supervisees expressing how they feel about the experience, and how they feel about working and sharing with the other group members. This is like Cole's "processing" step (2017, p. 4). Expressing feelings helps us to understand our responses to what happened in the group. This can be a challenging step to facilitate and may be easily overlooked.

Positive feelings are not so difficult to openly share. But when the group activity made a person feel anxious, embarrassed, or upset, it may be more difficult to express. Creating a safe group supervision space where people are encouraged to express **both positive and negative feelings can help us understand better what happened in the group** and why we behaved or reacted the way we did. If left unexpressed, any benefits of the group supervision could be over-ridden as a person can become overwhelmed by their feelings. However, if they are shared, then the supervisor can help to address them and help the person to understand the significance of those feelings (Cole, 2017). This is illustrated by Sarah's **Reflective Story (Box 7.8)**.

BOX 7.8

Reflective Story by Sarah Harvey: Processing feelings in group supervision

During a group supervision session I was facilitating, the discussion became focused on the work of occupational therapists in different practice settings. One group member (from setting A) discussed how they were thinking about changing their own assessment process, to mirror the work of occupational therapists from setting B, despite the fact it would not have been relevant to their practice setting.

The rest of the group members from setting A got quite excited about this idea. They started asking questions about how therapists in setting B worked and whether they could apply for funding to be trained to complete the same assessments.

During the group supervision, we examined why setting A therapists were so focused on the work of other people. It became evident that setting B's focus on standardised assessments made therapists in setting A feel anxious about how they were carrying out their assessments. From this comparison, they now believed they were using 'inferior' observational assessments.

When occupational therapists from setting A were asked to discuss their feelings further, one person stated that in other areas of their life, they often felt worried about missing out on experiences, and in this instance, they felt like they were missing out on training. Another person from setting A started talking about a lack of confidence and being anxious about making the right recommendations, stating that it would be easier to rely on a standardised assessment to validate their decisions.

Once the group had **explored** these anxieties and understood what was driving their conversations, therapists from setting A were able to refocus on the value of the chosen occupation-focused observational assessment and recognised what their team was already achieving. From this starting point, they were able to make meaningful plans to enhance their service provision, rather than following a path fuelled by their feelings of uncertainty.

When exploring what happened during the group, **underlying feelings may be recognised when the group goes 'off-task'**. In Sarah's story this happened when setting A therapists wanted to abandon their assessment process. Going off-task can also be seen when people **avoid talking**

about something that they find unsettling by changing the subject or focusing on something that is happening outside of the group. Or the group may flee from problematic conversations with the **use of humour**. You may also notice the group spending a lot of time discussing or ruminating on **things that are not within their control**, such as the way the larger service is run or funded. These situations could indicate that **the group is stuck, and you need to explore what they are feeling and why this might be**, before everyone can move on productively.

The other issues to pay attention to are **times when the group becomes conflicted**. At these times there may be struggles between people for power and control. Subgroups may form and the group may use this tactic to push through their ideas and dictate the conversation direction and any decisions made. This may happen when difficult subjects are discussed, or work is challenged. Wilfred Bion's Basic Assumption Groups Framework can be useful to further understand these group behaviours. This theory supports the idea that the patterns of observed group behaviours will be driven by the group's need to reduce anxiety and internal conflicts (French and Simpson, 2010). While it is beyond the scope of what we are discussing here, you may wish to consult other texts such as de Felice et al. (2019). But for now, we will move on to the final component of the Four Steps for Group Supervision, and how we can promote application of learning and action planning.

Application and next steps

Application and next steps are where the **cognitive learning aspects are addressed through the identification of general principles and consideration of how these can apply outside of the group** (Cole, 2017). General principles can be developed by looking for **patterns of responses** or common opinions of group members. For example, in Sarah's story, a general principle was having a shared anxiety about making sound decisions when conducting observational assessments. Areas of **disagreement** can also be considered a general principle. For example, some supervisees may share how much they learn from and enjoy taking students on placement, while others may see it as an additional challenge in an already overwhelming workload. General principles may also appear when you see the group's **energy rise** when discussing a certain topic. For example, when a topic generates spontaneous conversations and ideas, it is a sign that this area is important to the group (Cole, 2017).

Once the general principles are determined, the supervisor can present a few ideas succinctly (rather than recounting everything that happened in the group). The supervisor then **uses the general principles learned during the group and guides the conversation to how these can be applied outside of the group** (Cole, 2017). The aim is for each person to understand how the results of the group discussion could enhance their own work, learning, and/or self-management. Group problem-solving can also be encouraged as members help each other find ways to apply the new information. The group could potentially help monitor each other's progress between supervision sessions.

Finally, the supervisor summarises the important aspects of the group and everyone is thanked for their participation. This is to help reinforce the goals, content, and process of the group, including the emotional content. Supervisees are **encouraged to create a plan of a few actions** they intend to do from what they have learnt in the session. This could be anything from finding out more information, trying out a strategy, noting a new topic for supervision, or seeking out more opportunities to discuss and consolidate the topics raised. Asking supervisees **when they will carry out their actions** is one way of helping people to think about concrete next steps.

Your own time and commitments as a supervisor are also important to consider, and in the next section we will offer a few ideas to help you prepare for this role.

Taking on the role of group supervisor

As you take on the role of group supervisor, you may wish to spend some time doing your own personal reflection on the changing dynamics this role will have in your team (see **Box 7.9**). We also encourage you to consider the professional boundaries of your role and how your relationships may be impacted by becoming a group supervisor (or indeed any supervisor).

BOX 7.9

Reflective activities to help prepare for the role of group supervisor

- Using the Discussion-Based Reflective Model (Figure 7.3) with a trusted person or group, explore your past supervisory and leadership experiences, and how they might influence your group supervision style.
- If you feel you need to, seek out information about running groups and supervision strategies from the literature, more experienced colleagues, people from other disciplines, etc.
- Think about the needs of the supervisees potentially attending the group. Using Appendix 7.3 as a guide, create a draft plan of what the first group supervision session could look like.
- Look for professional development opportunities relating to supervision, leadership, and group working.
- If you are supervising a group outside your organisation, try to find out about the services provided and expertise required of the staff. Find out about local policies and procedures that guide work in their organisation.
- Find out about your potential group members, including their place within the organisation, who they report to, team structures, etc.
- Reflect on the current health, political, and economic climate, and how it impacts on service delivery.
- If you are worrying about your new role or feeling unsure about whether you have the skills to do it, raise it in your own supervision and/or with a trusted peer.

CRITICAL COMMENTARY

Why didn't we think of applying these ideas to supervision before?

As we embarked on writing this chapter, a question kept coming up for us: 'Why do we use so many skills in our therapy practice but don't always translate them into our supervision practices?' As you are reading this chapter, you may be thinking that you already apply your therapy knowledge, reasoning, and skills during supervision, and we do know many people are already doing this well. For us, it was through reflection on our own practices and many discussions that the extent of our therapy knowledge, reasoning, and skills, and their usefulness to supervision become apparent.

For example, through my teaching of students about group intervention methods I (Karina) use Cole's Seven Steps. It was only when thinking about how to explain a group supervision approach that I made the connection that we already had a useful way to think about the steps in running a group. I am reasonably convinced that if I were not writing a book, I would probably not have made the connection as I embarked on a group supervision session in my practice. However, once I thought about it and discussed it with my colleagues, it seemed obvious. So why didn't I think of it before?

From a learning and teaching perspective, we know that transferring knowledge between situations and contexts can be rare and unpredictable (Schell, 2018). Our literature frequently talks about the theory-to-practice gap, often in relation to students learning to become occupational therapy professionals (e.g. Thomas et al., 2017). Knowledge, skills, and strategies generally do not transfer well from one place to another (Brown et al., 1989) and thus perhaps we should not be surprised by our challenge even though we thought our student days were behind us. For us, it does open the next question: 'What else could we usefully apply to supervision that we haven't yet considered?'

SUMMARY

In this chapter we reviewed three areas familiar to occupational therapists in their work with people who access services and their potential application to supervision. Coaching, creativity, and group concepts were reviewed and ideas for how to practically apply them within a supervision framework discussed.

In the next chapter, we apply an appreciative, strengths-based perspective to supervision – particularly when tensions arise in the relationship. This continues our theme of applying what we know to supervisory practices for the safety and benefit of professionals and the public.

REFERENCES

Andersson, L., King, R., and Lalande, L. (2010) 'Dialogical mindfulness in supervision role-play', *Counselling and Psychotherapy Research*, 10, pp. 287–294. doi:10.1080/14733141003599500.

Bandura, A. (1977) *Social learning theory*. Englewood Cliffs: Prentice-Hall.

Bannigan, K. and Moores, A. (2009) 'A model of professional thinking: integrating reflective practice and evidence based practice', *Canadian Journal of Occupational Therapy*, 76(5), pp. 342–350. doi:10.1177/000841740907600505.

Bearman, S.K., Weisz, J.R., Chorpita, B.F., Hoagwood, K., Ward, A., Ugueto, A.M., and Bernstein, A. (2013) 'More practice, less preach? The role of supervision processes and therapist characteristics in EBP implementation', *Administration and Policy in Mental Health*, 40(6), pp. 518–529. doi:10.1007/s10488-013-0485-5.

Bennett-Levy, J., McManus, F., Westling, B.E., and Fennell, M. (2009) 'Acquiring and refining CBT skills and competencies: which training methods are perceived to be most effective?', *Behavioural and Cognitive Psychotherapy*, 37, pp. 571–583. doi:10.1017/S1352465809990270.

Brown, J.S., Collins, A., and Duguid, P. (1989) 'Situated cognition and the culture of learning', *Educational Researcher*, 18(1), pp. 32–42. doi:10.3102/0013189X018001032.

Cole, M.B. (2017) *Group dynamics in occupational therapy: the theoretical basis and practice application of group intervention*. 5th edn. Thorofare, NJ: Slack.

de Felice, G., De Vita, G., Bruni, A., Galimberti, A., Paoloni, G., Andreassi, S., and Giuliani, A. (2019) 'Group, basic assumptions and complexity science', *Group Analysis*, 52(1), pp. 3–22. doi:10.1177/0533316418791117.

Donald, E.J. and Carter, A. (2020) 'Overview of common group theories', in Killam, W.K., Carter, A., and Degges-White, S. (eds) *Group development and group leadership in student affairs*. London: Rowman & Littlefield Publishers, pp. 29–44.

French, R.B. and Simpson, P. (2010) 'The "work group": redressing the balance in Bion's *Experiences in groups*', *Human Relations*, 63(12), pp. 1859–1878. doi:10.1177/0018726710365091.

Graham, F. (2020) *Occupational Performance Coaching (OPC) session schedule*. Available at: https://www.otago.ac.nz/opc (Accessed: 21 July 2020).

Graham, F., Kennedy-Behr, A., and Ziviani, J. (2020) *Occupational Performance Coaching: a manual for practitioners and researchers*. Abingdon: Routledge.

Graham, F., Rodger, S., and Ziviani, J. (2010) 'Enabling occupational performance of children through coaching parents: three case reports', *Physical and Occupational Therapy in Pediatrics*, 30(1), pp. 4–15. doi:10.3109/01942630903337536.

Grant, A.M. (2011) 'Is it time to REGROW the GROW model? Issues related to teaching coaching session structures', *The Coaching Psychologist*, 7(2), pp. 118–126.

Iwama, M.K., Thomson, N.A., and Macdonald, R.M. (2009) 'The Kawa model: the power of culturally responsive occupational therapy', *Disability and Rehabilitation*, 31(14), pp. 1125–1135. doi:10.1080/09638280902773711.

King, G., Schwellnus, H., Servais. M., and Baldwin, P. (2019) 'Solution-focused coaching in pediatric rehabilitation: investigating transformative experiences and outcomes for families', *Physical and Occupational Therapy in Pediatrics*, 39(1), pp. 16–32. doi:10.1080/01942638.2017.1379457.

Milne, D.L., Sheikh, A.I., Pattison, S., and Wilkinson, A. (2011) 'Evidence-based training for clinical supervisors: a systematic review of 11 controlled studies', *The Clinical Supervisor*, 30, pp. 53–71. doi:10.1080/07325223.2011.564955.

Rodger, S. (2010). *Occupation-centred practice with children: a practical guide for occupational therapists*. Oxford: Wiley-Blackwell.

Rush, D.D. and Shelden, M.L. (2011) *The early childhood coaching handbook*. Baltimore, MD: Brookes Publishing Company.

Salinsky, J. (2009) *A very short introduction to Balint Groups*. Available at: https://balint.co.uk/about/introduction/ (Accessed: 3 November 2021).

Scaife, J. (2019) *Supervision in clinical practice: a practitioner's guide.* 3rd edn. Abingdon: Routledge.

Schell, J.W. (2018) 'Teaching for reasoning in higher education', in Schell, B.A.B. and Schell, J.W. (eds) *Clinical and professional reasoning in occupational therapy.* Philadelphia: Wolters Kluwer, pp. 417–437.

Thomas, A., Han, L., Osler, B.P., Turnbull, E.A., and Douglas, E. (2017) 'Students' attitudes and perceptions of teaching and assessment of evidence-based practice in an occupational therapy professional master's curriculum: a mixed methods study', *BMC Medical Education*, 17(1), pp. 1–11. doi:10.1186/s12909-017-0895-2.

Tuckman, B.W. (1965) 'Developmental sequence in small groups', *Psychological Bulletin*, 63, pp. 384–399. doi:10.1037/h0022100.

Tuckman, B.W. and Jensen, M.A. (1977) 'Stages of small-group development revisited', *Group and Organizational Studies*, 2, pp. 419–427. doi:10.1177/105960117700200404.

Whitmore, J. (1992) *Coaching for performance: a practical guide to growing your own skills.* London: Nicholas Brealey Publishing.

Appendix 7.1: PROPER Coaching for Supervision guidance template

1. Example questions to establish the supervisee's PRIORITY for discussion	
• Tell me about your workday/something you are working on. • What would you like to focus on? Why is this important right now? • What would it look like if it were going really well? • If you were able to change anything, what would it be? • What change would have the biggest impact on you / your colleagues / the people who use your services? • How much energy do you have for this now?	Notes:
2. Example questions to establish the supervisee's REALITY of the situation	
• What happens now? What have you tried; how did it go? • What have you thought about trying? • What supports do you have; what has worked so far? • What challenges do you expect to encounter?	Notes:
3. Example questions to establish the OPPORTUNITIES for change	
• What are some things you think you could do to reach your goal? Do not worry about how practical or good they are at this stage. What are the pros and cons of each option? • If you were at your most resourceful (or someone you feel is more able to deal with this) what would you/they be able to do? • Would you like me to share some ideas/information?	Notes:

4. EXAMPLE QUESTIONS TO ESTABLISH THE SUPERVISEE'S PLAN FOR CHANGE	
• From the list created, what would you try first? Next? • What makes this option a good choice? • What alternatives could there be to your plan? • When will you start?	**Notes:**
5. EXAMPLE QUESTIONS TO EVALUATE HOW THE SUPERVISEE FEELS ABOUT THEIR PLAN	
• How confident are you on a scale of 1–10 about doing your plan? What would make it a 9 or 10? • How can I help? What do you need from me?	**Notes:**
6. EXAMPLE QUESTIONS WHEN REVIEWING GOALS IN A FOLLOW-UP SESSION	
• Is this goal still a priority for you? • What happened when you attempted the plan? • Is there anything you wish to change? • What did you learn about yourself as a person/professional?	**Notes:**

Appendix 7.2: PROPER Coaching for Supervision documentation template

Date:	
People present:	
Format: (online / face-to-face / group / peer)	
Priority topics discussed	
Reality of what is happening now	
Opportunities identified that could lead to change	
Plan for what will be achieved and how it will happen I will [achieve something], in [this context/situation], to this [extent/quality/frequency], by this date. To do this I will: [list steps to meet the goal]	
Evaluate on a scale of 1–10 how confident I feel about doing this plan and what else could help	
Review in the next session what remains important, what happened since last session and what next	
Signed by supervisor and supervisee	

Appendix 7.3: Four Steps for Group Supervision guidance template

1. WELCOME	
• Warm-up • Setting the mood and expectations • Focus of the supervision	**Notes:**
2. MAIN ACTIVITY	
• Choice of activity • Hear from each person about what was done • Acknowledge involvement and contribution	**Notes:**
3. EXPLORATION	
• Expressing feelings about the activity and others • Can be positive or negative	**Notes:**
4. APPLICATION AND NEXT STEPS	
• Summarise a few key general principles from the main activity and exploration • Encourage supervisees to think about how learning can be applied to their work • Supervisees to commit to any actions • Thanks to all	**Notes:**

 Appendix 7.4: Group reflection guidance template

1. DESCRIBE	
• What happened? • What did you do? • What did others do? • What was the outcome?	**Notes:**
2. SEEK DIFFERENT PERSPECTIVES	
• Frame the situation using a professional model; what do you notice? • Think about the focus of the situation (e.g., communication, reasoning); what does the literature say about this? • What are others suggesting? • What ideas did you not notice before?	**Notes:**
3. MAKE SENSE	
• How do you feel now about what happened? • How did others react? • Why do you think this happened this way? • What do you now understand about the experience?	**Notes:**

4. Plan and 5. Document	

• What would happen if:
   o I kept doing it this way?
   o I made some adjustments? What would I do differently?
   o I sought out other perspectives?
   o I changed my practice? What will change?
   o I did some research? What do I want to find out?
• Note any new insights discovered or what has been reinforced for you.
• Keep a record of any plans and set a date to review.
	Notes:

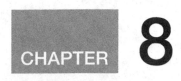

Working through tensions in supervision

Anita Volkert and Karina Dancza

With contributions from Stephanie Tempest, Shamala Thilarajah, Sarah Harvey, Suhailah Mohamed, Wong Su Ren, and Esther Yuen Ling Tai

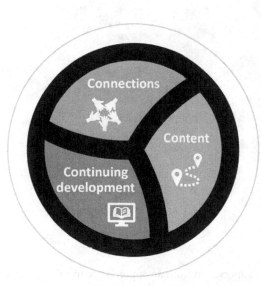

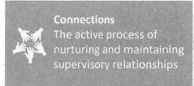

Connections
The active process of nurturing and maintaining supervisory relationships

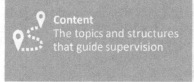

Content
The topics and structures that guide supervision

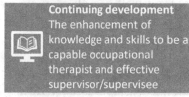

Continuing development
The enhancement of knowledge and skills to be a capable occupational therapist and effective supervisor/supervisee

DOI: 10.4324/9781003092544-8

CHAPTER INTENTIONS

In this chapter, we invite you to:

- Explore three common tensions that present in supervision
- Consider a range of practical, appreciative, strengths-based approaches to work through common tensions in supervision
- Relate the practical approaches to your context to identify elements to transfer into your own practice.

CHAPTER HIGHLIGHTS

- Common tensions that arise in supervision
- Using an appreciative, strengths-based approach
- Tension 1: Support versus performance evaluation
- Tension 2: Power and hierarchy
- Tension 3: Supervisor or supervisee appears to over- or underestimate their own abilities
- Critical commentary: Are we ignoring challenges and problems?

CHAPTER RESOURCES

Figures

- Figure 8.1 The Appreciative Inquiry Cycle
- Figure 8.2 Strengths-Based Self-Evaluation Tool for Supervisors
- Figure 8.3 Johari Window

Table

- Table 8.1 Places to seek external supervision

Boxes

- Box 8.1 Generative questions for use in supervision from an appreciative inquiry perspective
- Box 8.2 Benefits of an appreciative, strengths-based approach to supervision
- Box 8.3 Illustrative example: Chris and Jo – the tension of a dual role as supervisor and line manager
- Box 8.4 Illustrative example: Chris and Jo – using the Appreciative Inquiry Cycle to work through the tension
- Box 8.5 Applying an appreciative, strengths-based approach
- Box 8.6 Reflective Story by Wong Su Ren and Esther Yuen Ling Tai: Setting up group mentoring

- Box 8.7 Editor's Reflective Story: Looking for supervision outside your organisation
- Box 8.8 Reflective Story by Sarah Harvey: Realities of power and hierarchy in supervision
- Box 8.9 Illustrative example: When you have done all you can as a supervisor
- Box 8.10 Reflective Story by Suhailah Mohamed: Reframing a challenging situation
- Box 8.11 Illustrative example: Pin Xiu and Kennedy – the tension of appearing to overestimate abilities
- Box 8.12 Illustrative example: Pin Xiu and Kennedy – changing the narrative
- Box 8.13 Common areas of accommodation in the workplace
- Box 8.14 Reflecting on your own supervisory needs

Appendices

- Appendix 8.1 Strengths-Based Self-Evaluation Tool for Supervisors guidance template
- Appendix 8.2 Reflection activity using the Johari Window

COMMON TENSIONS THAT ARISE IN SUPERVISION

As supervision is likely to feature throughout our careers, it is anticipated that at some point everyone will experience a tension associated with being a supervisor or supervisee. In this chapter, we want to encourage open conversations about tensions and consider ways of working through them. We harness the 3Cs for Effective Supervision and propose an appreciative, strengths-based approach to explore some common tensions. Through describing how we approach these tensions we hope that you find useful strategies to apply in your own situation. The three tensions we will illustrate relate to:

- the tension that can arise between adopting a **supportive approach and the need to evaluate and manage performance** in supervision
- **issues of power**, including but not limited to hierarchy, culture, gender, ability, class, and belief, and
- when the supervisor or supervisee **appears to over- or underestimate their abilities**, or there is a different perspective of their capabilities.

To begin, we will offer a brief overview of what we mean by an appreciative, strengths-based approach.

USING AN APPRECIATIVE, STRENGTHS-BASED APPROACH

The foundation of an appreciative, strengths-based approach is the value placed on the capacity, skills, knowledge, connections, and potential the person brings into supervision. Supervision focuses on how the supervisee can develop their capability and continuously improve their performance as they advance in work or study. Appreciative, strengths-based perspectives are a good fit for this purpose, as they aim to foster growth by focusing on the vision of where one wants to go.

An appreciative, strengths-based approach (or some may refer to it as an appreciative inquiry [Cooperrider and Srivastva, 1987; Cooperrider, 2013]) involves asking **generative questions**, which stimulate curiosity and creativity in working towards the defined vision or goal. Generative questions help people think about old problems or issues in new ways (Stavros et al., 2018). They keep the focus on **what could be possible**, and by doing so help both supervisor and supervisee come up with options for what to do next that they previously had not considered. Examples of generative questions that may be helpful to use in supervision are in **Box 8.1**.

BOX 8.1

Generative questions for use in supervision from an appreciative inquiry perspective

- What is it about you that will make this happen?
- What else do you need for it to succeed? Where can we find that?
- Imagine you were doing this work exactly how you thought it needed to be done? What would change for the better?
- How have you seen (a respected colleague) handle this?
- What is one thing you could do differently to make a positive difference?

This positive focus, permission to dream about one's ideal outcome then taking practical steps to achieve the dream, is what makes an appreciative, strengths-based perspective particularly useful when the supervisor or supervisee feels 'stuck' and needs to renew their own energy to find a way forward. While there is a range of appreciative, strengths-based perspectives, we have found **the Appreciative Inquiry Cycle** (Cooperrider et al., 2008) a useful summary **(Figure 8.1)**.

In the Appreciative Inquiry Cycle, the first step is to **Define** the situation or context of interest (which may present as an issue, tension, or problem); **Discovery** is where you find out what is currently happening; **Dream** is what the ideal situation might look like; **Design** is where you see what needs to happen to move from the existing situation to the ideal one; and **Delivery** is where you plan and seek commitment for change.

Adopting an appreciative, strengths-based approach does not mean discounting or ignoring the problems that people bring into their supervisory sessions. As Graybeal (2001, p. 234) explains, "the identification of strengths is not the antithesis of the identification of problems. Instead, it is a large part of the solution." You may find that using a deficits approach, where you focus on what's going wrong and on improving perceived weaknesses, works at times. Acknowledging both

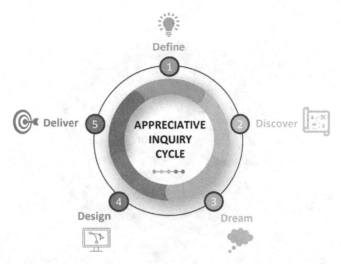

FIGURE 8.1 The Appreciative Inquiry Cycle (adapted from Cooperrider et al., 2008)

approaches is important, although evidence suggests that it would be useful to redress the balance between the more dominant deficits approach and an appreciative, strengths-based perspective (Fialkov and Haddad, 2012).

Ultimately, an appreciative, strengths-based approach means that both supervisor and supervisee are working together to produce what is needed to create positive change, rather than, for example, the supervisee being a passive recipient of expert advice from a supervisor (Rapp et al., 2008; Berg, 2009). It has the potential to offer alternative perspectives and we invite you to consider these highlighted in **Box 8.2**.

BOX 8.2

Benefits of an appreciative, strengths-based approach to supervision

An appreciative, strengths-based approach can:

- create significant change (Cojocaru, 2010)
- create an atmosphere which promotes safe and positive inquiry and questioning
- enable powerful role modelling
- assist supervisees and supervisors to link emotions with learning (Schreibman and Chilton, 2012)
- inject hope into the supervisory relationship and process, and
- move supervision from telling it like it is to telling it as it may become (Srivastva et al., 1990, cited in Gonzalez, 1997).

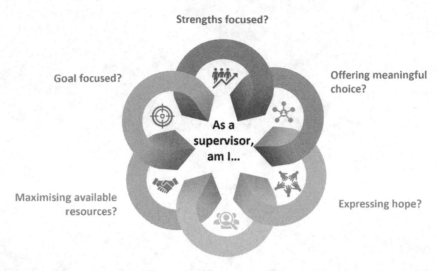

Strengths focused?

Goal focused?

Offering meaningful choice?

As a supervisor, am I...

Maximising available resources?

Expressing hope?

Making strengths explicit?

FIGURE 8.2 Strengths-Based Self-Evaluation Tool for Supervisors (adapted from Rapp et al., 2008)

If you are a supervisor thinking about your own supervisory style and how to include a more appreciative, strengths-based approach, a useful place to begin is to think about your own strengths and the aspects of your character that have served you well in your career so far. The **Strengths-Based Self-Evaluation Tool for Supervisors** (adapted from Rapp et al., 2008) shown in **Figure 8.2** offers a framework for considering your strengths so you can make explicit use of them in supervision. **Appendix 8.1 offers some additional reflective questions** to help explore your supervisory strengths.

Using frameworks focused on strengths, as well as areas for development, encourages a holistic and balanced approach to issues and tensions that may arise within a supervisory relationship (Davys and Beddoe, 2020). In the next section we will explore three common tensions that may arise in supervision, and how we use an appreciative, strengths-based approach to work through them.

TENSION 1: SUPPORT VERSUS PERFORMANCE EVALUATION

One of the most common tensions in supervision happens when the supervisor occupies a dual role (Mette et al., 2017). Being a line manager and in charge of tasks such as work allocation, approval of leave requests, performance appraisal or review, etc. can potentially conflict with the supportive and professional development functions of a supervisor. The reality is, however, that in many organisations supervisors often hold both roles simultaneously. This tension can be particularly acute if the supervisor is asked to formally performance manage their supervisee, i.e. closely monitor actions of an underperforming supervisee to bring them up to a minimum standard so they can remain employed in that role. The illustrative example in **Box 8.3**, shares a story of Jo who is a supervisor and line manager to Chris, and how a tension is brewing in their relationship.

BOX 8.3

Illustrative example: Chris and Jo – the tension of a dual role as supervisor and line manager

Jo is supervising Chris, a person with two years' graduate experience. Jo is Chris' line manager and supervisor but does not work in the same team or specialised area as Chris. Chris has a separate team leader who monitors some aspects of his work. Chris is well liked in his team and in the wider organisation and has an outgoing personality. However, Jo has received complaints from the team that Chris doesn't always meet deadlines. Chris' team leader and colleagues are reluctant to bring this up with him and Jo has been asked to address this issue in supervision. If left, the issue will likely compound, and become an issue for the organisation, and a performance management issue for Chris. Chris has not raised meeting deadlines as a concern in supervision, tending to focus on either very specific problems and questions, or more general personal and professional development.

The scenario of Jo and Chris may sound familiar to you as either the supervisor knowing there is an issue but perhaps not sure how to raise it; or as a supervisee wanting to do your best but not sure how asking for help would reflect on you. Whilst some of the supervision models that we refer to in Chapter 1 such as Proctor's three functions of supervision suggest a link between supportive, managerial, and educative areas, what to do when tensions arise is less well articulated. Thus, when major tensions between support and evaluation arise, other models may be required to help us structure how to approach the situation, such as the Appreciative Inquiry Cycle (Cooperrider et al., 2008) outlined in **Figure 8.1**. We will follow the story of Jo and Chris as Jo uses this approach to raise the issue of Chris' performance (**Box 8.4**).

BOX 8.4

Illustrative example: Chris and Jo – using the Appreciative Inquiry Cycle to work through the tension

DEFINE what is happening now

Initially, Jo gently asks Chris about case and workload management. Chris moves on quickly from this topic and asks about something else that is unrelated. Jo redirects Chris and explains that an issue has been raised from within the team. Chris then admits to finding it hard to keep up with the work, feeling caught in a downward spiral.

Chris was embarrassed at first when the topic was raised by Jo. He hadn't wanted to lose face in supervision by admitting to not coping. Chris reflected that he had responded by ignoring the problem and hoping it would go away. Chris admitted that he had been feeling so stressed that he had been having trouble sleeping and was considering leaving the job.

As the conversation progressed, Chris felt a profound sense of relief that the problem was now in the open, although he remained embarrassed about seeming not able to cope. Jo and Chris agree to work on workload management in supervision.

DISCOVER what is working well, strengths and capabilities

Jo and Chris then spend time exploring past high points – times in Chris' career when he was managing his workload well, exploring the strengths and capabilities that contributed to this. This was a positive, energetic, and productive conversation. They identified key strengths, including commitment and perseverance, a desire to do a good job, and Chris' natural good humour and friendliness.

DREAM about the potential for change

Together, they imagined how the current situation would look if these strengths and capabilities could be tapped into, and another high point created. They considered the goals again and thought about how these strengths and capabilities will help make progress towards them.

DESIGN the next steps to get closer to the dream

Jo and Chris focused on some immediate steps. They worked out a detailed weekly schedule, listing direct work with people accessing services and administrative time, along with clear rest breaks to re-energise. Chris' schedule would be busy, but they tapped into his commitment, perseverance, and desire to do a good job. They also considered what could be appropriately delegated on the task list, and Chris used his good relationships with other team members to achieve this, as well as to receive support as Chris started to become more open and ask for help from team members.

DELIVER on the plan

Jo and Chris used supervision to refine the plan and turn these steps into ongoing habits. Three months later Chris' team leader contacted Jo to say how marked the improvement was in Chris' workload management. The team had also reportedly noticed the changes. Six months later, Chris receives a highly positive performance review, and is no longer thinking about leaving the organisation.

We invite you to take some time to reflect on the illustrative example of Chris and Jo. **Box 8.5** offers some prompt questions that may help. You might want to make some notes on your thoughts and potentially raise them in a conversation with your own supervisor or trusted peer.

BOX 8.5

Applying an appreciative, strengths-based approach

- What are your initial thoughts and feelings after reading the illustrative story?
- Have you had similar experiences from your own professional life, as either (or both) supervisor and supervisee? If you have, you might want to consider your own story and even write it out.
- Would an appreciative, strengths-based approach have made a difference to how your own experience played out? If so, what might have been different?

Chris and Jo were able to navigate the support and avoid close performance management in the earlier example. While this is ideal, things may not always be so successful. In many occupational therapy services, supervision consists of one supervisor to one supervisee. While there is nothing wrong with this arrangement, when the supervisor is also the line manager, it can create tensions. We introduced in Chapter 3 the idea of a portfolio of supervision, and this is something we will again return to. A portfolio of supervision can include this common supervisor-to-supervisee arrangement, but other opportunities could include group supervision with peers or colleagues, supervision from other professionals, or seeking an additional supervisor outside of your organisation.

The following **Reflective Story** by Wong Su Ren and Esther Yuen Ling Tai shares how an acute hospital created a new support structure for supervisors starting out in their supervisory roles **(Box 8.6)**. This consisted of a group mentoring programme run by Su Ren and Esther, two experienced occupational therapists and supervisors.

BOX 8.6

Reflective Story by Wong Su Ren and Esther Yuen Ling Tai: Setting up group mentoring

In our acute hospital setting, a study was conducted on perceptions of value-based occupational therapy (Wong et al., 2021). The occupational therapists in the study highlighted that additional mentoring and guidance were desired, especially for those who had recently taken on a role as a supervisor. The study results triggered an exploration of setting up a mentoring programme to meet the needs of these new supervisors.

We started with a discussion between Su Ren and Esther as we both were interested and thought our skill sets complemented each other. As Su Ren comes from a life coaching and mental health background, she offered in-depth coaching and practical interpersonal skills to manage various situations. Esther comes from an educational background and emphasised the concept of growing and learning in a mentoring relationship. Moreover, we engage in peer mentoring between ourselves, which allowed us to continually reflect on our own knowledge and skills.

We first sent a survey to invite newly promoted supervisors to indicate their interest in group mentoring; we recruited a total of seven people as a closed group. In the survey they expressed that they wished to focus on understanding their role in supervision, how to deal with challenging situations, and interpersonal skills. As a group, we decided on bimonthly hour-long group mentoring. Each session started with 10–15 minutes of sharing on topics of interest, while the rest of time was set aside to bring up scenarios that they were facing, share ideas, and address some of the challenges and pitfalls in supervision. We also offered the group the opportunity for individual mentoring. Initially, due to COVID-19 restrictions, the sessions needed to be online but where possible, we started having face-to-face sessions as we felt it was important for relationship development. We decided to pilot this for one year.

We created a shared group notebook for people to describe their goals and to write down any interesting issues that they wanted to discuss during the sessions. We placed it in a central but secure location. Su Ren, Esther, and the seven mentees could access, write, and read through the one-year group journey reflected in the notebook.

Initially, we thought this book would provide a sense of group identity and a common point of reflection. As an unexpected benefit, it also allowed time and space for people who were more comfortable with anonymous expression to write down their challenges. It offered a safe space for those who were struggling and not yet comfortable to share their thoughts, ideas, or stories verbally in the group.

During each session, we would pick examples from the notebook to discuss. We noticed similarities between the issues and challenges, such as what it meant to be a supervisor, difficulties in differentiating between being 'friends' or 'supervisor', and how to respond to supervisees who were not coping and how to approach them to offer help. We found the notebook was key in kickstarting many of the discussions during the group.

As we continued the sessions, the content morphed into what was necessary for the mentees and we encouraged them to actively take the discussion where it needed to go. We left the last session for open-ended discussions, as people felt more and more comfortable to verbalise their struggles and scenarios.

Su Ren and Esther's story illustrates how they were able to create opportunities for the therapists to use multiple supervisors within the organisation to complement their portfolio. In other situations, it may be that looking outside the organisation for these different opinions is valuable. In the following **Editor's Reflective Story**, Anita shares how she sought an external coach to help her decide on her next career move (**Box 8.7**).

BOX 8.7

Editor's Reflective Story: Looking for supervision outside your organisation

At a mid-point in my career, I (Anita) found myself in the position of having two options – of remaining within my current organisation in a role I enjoyed but felt I had outgrown or moving sideways to a role which did not offer a promotion, more money, or an easier commute, but I knew the supervisor and I was excited by the opportunities they would create for me. I did not know what to do, so I sought external coaching to help me make the decision.

I found the external coaching experience very useful. The coach listened, reflected my thoughts back to me, and most importantly, helped me consider the options more lightly – after all, what was the worst that could happen? I made my decision and accepted the new position (even with the reservations I had) and found that as I had suspected, I did indeed flourish in the new supervisory environment. It was what I needed at that time, and the coach helped me to trust my instincts and abilities in decision making much more, as well as helping me dispense with overthinking and second-guessing myself.

Anita's story highlights that at a certain timepoint, she found meeting with someone outside of her organisation enabled her to make decisions about what was best for her and her career. If you find yourself in a similar situation, there is a range of places to seek external supervision, and we have outlined a few in **Table 8.1**. In addition, you can also look beyond occupational therapy as there is **value in seeking supervisory perspectives from outside of our profession**. Always consider an informal conversation to find out more about the work

TABLE 8.1 Places to seek external supervision

NATIONAL PROFESSIONAL ASSOCIATIONS
Associations may collate and publish lists of accredited or approved supervisors

Advantages
- Assurance that supervisor expertise has been reviewed and approved by an independent source
- Easy resource to access if you are a member of a professional association
- May offer regional groups to connect with at a local level

(Continued)

TABLE 8.1 (Continued)

Disadvantages
- May need to be paid member to access resources
- Limits the potential pool of supervisors to only those from the same profession
- Resources may not be regularly updated

SPECIAL INTEREST GROUPS / COMMUNITIES OF PRACTICE
Provides access to practitioners who may be interested in offering supervision

Advantages
- Joining a group enables you to have formal or informal interactions with a potential supervisor prior to engaging them. This offers some insight into the attributes and expertise of potential supervisors
- Potential for you to create peer or group supervision opportunities

Disadvantages
- May take some time to get known in the group
- May feel intimidating to approach experts to determine if they offer supervision
- It could be difficult to find relevant groups to join

SOCIAL MEDIA GROUPS
Social media platforms and their use are constantly changing, and you may wish to create a professional profile separate from your personal profile

Advantages
- Provides potential access to a wide range of people
- Free and accessible for most people

Disadvantages
- Will be limited to digitally active people which could influence the direction of the conversations
- May be difficult to identify potential supervisors
- Some people may not respond to you if they do not know you (fear of scams), so it could be time-consuming to find someone suitable

PROFESSIONAL COACH AND/OR MENTORS
These are private businesses that offer fee-for-service supervision

Advantages
- Choice is available through independent websites including occupational therapists who also qualify as coaches
- Could provide different perspectives from working outside of health and social care
- Potential to find skilled supervisors as it is their core business rather than an add-on to their regular job

Disadvantages
- Variation in the services provided
- Quality will need to be independently considered
- Prices will vary

UNIVERSITY/EDUCATION INSTITUTIONS
Academic faculty may offer supervision as a fee-for-service or part of their role

Advantages
- You may already have a relationship with a faculty member from your professional education
- They could offer practice, educational, and research perspectives

Disadvantages
- Faculty may have fluctuating availability as they fit in supervision around their existing workload
- Systems for external supervision may not be set up within the university

the external supervisor does, their background experience, and what they feel they can offer you in terms of your development. The conversation should be focused on identifying your needs and the ways they can you support you – not on the supervisor pressuring you to buy their service.

TENSION 2: POWER AND HIERARCHY

Power is a major dynamic in any supervisory relationship. We have a long history of a hierarchical structure to many workplaces, and this plays out in our conception of, and expectations of, supervision. Supervisors can feel a weight of expectation to come up with answers, be the 'experts', and be right in their decisions. Supervisors can also feel frustrated or disappointed if supervisees choose not to follow their 'good' advice. Supervisors' own internal feelings of self-doubt may also result in either overcompensating with too much control, or undercompensating with too little input. The following **Reflective Story** by Sarah Harvey illustrates the tensions that can arise when the realities of power and hierarchical structures impact on supervision (**Box 8.8**).

BOX 8.8

Reflective Story by Sarah Harvey: Realities of power and hierarchy in supervision

There were times when supervision did not work. As an occupational therapist fresh out of university, I was allocated an occupational therapy technical instructor/assistant to supervise. While this was a way of increasing my skills as an occupational therapist and expanding my experience, when I look back it does seem a little unfair to the technical instructor who had worked in mental health for over 20 years. At that time, my mental health experience consisted of a 12-week placement and a six-month preceptorship.

Enthusiastically I structured my sessions with reflective space, goals, and career development ideas. The supervisee was fantastic at talking for hours, and I thought we were getting on very well. This was until I heard the term "jumped-up university student" being used to describe me, and I was firmly put back in my place. I learned the hard way what an honest conversation should look like, and if I had had the confidence, it would have probably been wise to discuss how the supervisee felt about having a newly qualified supervisor before we started working together. A lesson learned (the hard way).

Another time later in my career I experienced the same situation but this time I had more experience than my allocated supervisor. The supervisor appeared to cope with this disparity on the surface, but what they did was an increasing form of micromanagement. The supervisor attempted to demonstrate their own skills by focusing on how I could be more efficient and effective in my work. On reflection I think this was probably because they were worried or even threatened by my experience. Consequently, it stifled our relationship; there was no ability to be creative, to analyse cases, or reflect on practice. Instead, it just became the supervisor instructing me what to do and I was to follow.

Facilitating an open, supportive, and honest environment is a **key responsibility of a supervisor**. Establishing this safe space goes a long way toward preventing unhelpful tensions and conflicts, and it paves the way for personal and professional growth (as we introduced in chapters 1 and 4). A supervisor does not necessarily have to have more experience than a supervisee, or be higher up the hierarchy, as one of the primary aims of supervision is not to tell others what to do, but to facilitate learning, growth, and development. Helpful approaches are **being transparent, making expectations clear at the outset, and beginning well** – discussing and planning for tensions before they happen (please also see Chapter 5 and creating the supervisory arrangement).

Supervisory power manifests itself as supervisors may be able to make recommendations in relation to the supervisee for promotion, enable future career opportunities, provide references, and have access to insider knowledge within an organisation. As we have seen in the story of Chris, it is possible that, as the supervisee, they may experience anxiety about their performance, but due to the power imbalance feel unable to share their fears and concerns openly due to the potential effect it may have on performance appraisal/review and future career prospects.

As an alternative perspective, we invite you to read our next illustrative example written as an honest account from the perspective of a supervisor **(Box 8.9)**. In this example, the supervisor acknowledges and uses their power to create opportunities for a supervisee but struggles when the supervisee is not able to successfully use those opportunities.

BOX 8.9

Illustrative example: When you have done all you can as a supervisor

Being a supervisor is not an easy experience. There are times when, despite your best efforts to be positive and supportive, the changes you see in a supervisee just don't meet the minimum standards required or come at a pace that is acceptable. One example of this was when a supervisee had issues with public speaking (something that was required in their role), and I admit that I struggled to sustain my positive attitude. Recognising a hidden talent for creativity and innovation in the supervisee, I created opportunities for the supervisee to engage with and present to stakeholders from different backgrounds. However, after a few presentations that did not go well, and a separate performance management issue being brought to my attention, I started wondering if the supervisee would be able to meet expected standards in this role.

Another thought that also crossed my mind was how, by using my own contacts to create opportunities for the supervisee, it could potentially reflect negatively on my own reputation and damage the goodwill I had created. On reflection, I may have subconsciously started altering the opportunities I created for the supervisee to minimise the potentially negative impact their below-expected performance had on others. I did persevere with the aim of developing self-reflection in the supervisee to unearth the reasons for the performance issues. However, over time the pattern repeated, and it was difficult for me to continue as I felt I had given as much as I could.

At this point I felt it was time to bring our supervisory relationship to a close and was working through how to do this in my own supervision. Coincidently, this happened around the time that I was moving in my own career, so I discontinued my role as supervisor, honestly with some sense of relief.

You may relate to this illustrative example and how despite best efforts, there are times when the supervisory relationship has run its course and it benefits all involved to move on. Seeking your own support as a supervisor is important to manage our own emotions about any major tension in supervision. To help you think about your own situation, we invite you to take some time to reflect on this story using the prompt questions previously suggested in Box 8.5. You may like to add to your previous notes and again raise any points of interest in your own supervision or with a trusted peer.

To use strategies effectively to work through tensions in supervision requires consideration of our own attitudes and beliefs. When we tune into ourselves, we can also become aware of potentially different viewpoints, values, and experiences and recognise what could be a shared perspective and what we might see in very different ways. We introduced these ideas in Chapter 1, when we described the Queer People of Color Resilience-Based Model (Singh and Chun, 2010), the Cyclical Model of White Awareness (Ryde, 2009), and the Identity Conscious Supervisory Approach (Brown et al., 2020). Awareness of potentially differing beliefs can inform our supervision approaches and communication styles. For example, Tsui (2004) described the supervisory culture of social workers in Hong Kong as 'loose', with few formal documents used such as agendas or contracts, and tensions are avoided through the cultural dominance of 'face'.

Unfortunately, there are times where the power and control issues that lie within supervisory relationships move into the realm of toxicity, narcissism, and abuse. Carlson et al. (2012) explored abusive supervisory relationships, and their negative impact on supervisee home and family life, and burnout. None of us think we are the kind of person who would do this; but this is not something we can simply assume. We may not be fully aware of the impact our communication style and approach to supervision have on others.

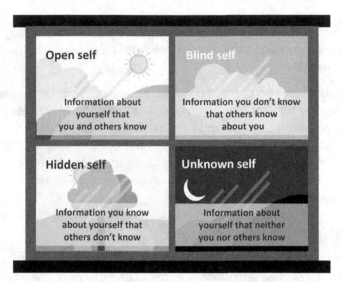

FIGURE 8.3 Johari Window (adapted from Luft and Ingham, 1955)

Being critically reflective, revisiting ideas of power and hierarchy frequently, and ensuring your own support and development are ways to monitor and even mitigate potentially harmful supervision. **Figure 8.3**, **the Johari Window** (Luft and Ingham, 1955) may be a familiar reflection tool for you. This can be a useful way to become aware of the aspects of ourselves we are blind to, and don't know about ourselves. Considering it by yourself or sharing it in your own supervision for discussion and self-reflection, could be useful whatever your level of supervisory experience. **Appendix 8.2** offers a Johari Window reflective activity with ideas on how it could be used.

Our next **Reflective Story** in this section by Suhailah Mohamed illustrates the impact that reflection and reframing using an appreciative, strengths-based perspective can have on tensions that arise in supervision (**Box 8.10**). Suhailah deliberately chose to view a difficult event in a positive light, and by considering different viewpoints she was able to consolidate what happened in a way that was not immediately obvious. **Reframing** (Masters, 1992) is a good approach for helping us move from a fixed to a growth mindset, and you may like to revisit this in our Chapter 2 discussions. For now, let's hear from Suhailah.

BOX 8.10

Reflective Story by Suhailah Mohamed: Reframing a challenging situation

The situation

In my first role as a registered occupational therapist, I supervised two occupational therapy assistants.

The arrangement was for me to facilitate clinical and managerial supervision and raise any concerns to the clinical team lead as needed. Having come into occupational therapy from a career in health and social care recruitment, I felt able to apply supervisory skills from previous employment to the role.

One of my supervisees was a highly experienced therapy assistant, keen to pursue funded pre-registration occupational therapy study. With their consent, I sought advice from the clinical lead about suitable professional development opportunities that would further their career goals.

In the months that followed, the supervisee went directly to the clinical lead to discuss their professional development opportunities. They then presented me with information they gathered, and actions agreed with the clinical lead during our supervision sessions.

My initial thoughts as the supervisor

I felt like our supervision sessions had established a reciprocated, open, trusting, and encouraging relationship, so when this situation happened, I was surprised. I honestly felt undermined as a supervisor and disappointed. I initially interpreted the supervisee's actions as them going above me because of my lack of knowledge about professional development opportunities and processes. However, I acknowledged that the information the supervisee was seeking was beyond my knowledge base at the time and I learned a lot from it.

Reframing the situation and seeing it from the supervisee's perspective

The situation reinforced for me the power of the hierarchal organisational structure that I was working within. I realised that because the decisions about professional development were often made at higher levels of practice, the process was lengthy. I could see that my supervisee may have become impatient and thought it easier to approach the clinical lead directly.

It was also possible that the supervisee believed they were being helpful and saving me the task of raising the request with the lead. They also knew that they weren't my only supervisee and that I had a growing workload, so they may have been considering my other work commitments. Additionally, they had worked within the team for longer than I and had established relationships with the team leads. It probably felt natural to approach them with requests.

In this reflective story, the situation could have escalated into a toxic outcome if Suhailah responded with anger or reacted by increasing control within the supervisory relationship. Instead, Suhailah uses an appreciative-style reflection to better understand the motivations of her supervisee. She realises that the supervisee may not have been bypassing her, or finding their supervision sessions unhelpful or useless, but instead being considerate of Suhailah's workload. This helpful **reframe** meant that Suhailah's response to the situation came from a place of compassion and concern for her supervisee. We invite you now to take some time to reflect on the stories by Sarah and Suhailah and consider aspects that may be helpful for your own situation. The questions in Box 8.5 from earlier may help.

Overall, when there is a commitment to exploring hierarchical and power structures within the supervisory relationship, rather than just use the structures to exercise authority (Falender, 2009), real change and development can happen for both the supervisor and supervisee, but also the systems we work within. In our next section we will explore another tension that happens when a supervisor or supervisee appears to over- or underestimate their own abilities.

TENSION 3: SUPERVISOR OR SUPERVISEE APPEARS TO OVER- OR UNDERESTIMATE THEIR OWN ABILITIES

When people hold a different view of their abilities from what a reasonable external evaluator may see, it is likely to create a tension in supervision. While we are not saying everyone must hold the same view of a person's abilities, when significant discrepancies occur it may impact on a person's safety to do the job, success in their career, or relationships within the workplace (and potentially many other areas too). In the following illustrative example of Pin Xiu (supervisor) and Kennedy (supervisee) we share a situation we have found ourselves in during our careers and describe one way of approaching this tension (**Box 8.11**).

BOX 8.11

Illustrative example: Pin Xiu and Kennedy – the tension of appearing to overestimate abilities

Pin Xiu recently joined a medium-sized organisation as a middle-level manager, and was immediately asked to supervise Kennedy, a recent graduate occupational therapist. Kennedy's line manager had requested this additional supervision, as they were finding Kennedy difficult to manage. Pin Xiu was informed in the handover that Kennedy was "arrogant" and "over-confident" and had been getting team members off-side as a result. Pin Xiu decided to go in with an open mind and use an appreciative, strengths-based approach. She also reviewed some literature about communication and learning styles of different generations in practice now.

In Pin Xiu's first meeting with Kennedy, they set up their supervision relationship and agreements, and finished with an open discussion about the experience of working in the organisation. Kennedy did not feel that her prior experience of supervision had been useful and suggested that she was more knowledgeable than her supervisor. Kennedy also mentioned that the organisation had a "funny culture" and that she didn't feel part of the team.

Pin Xiu chose not to focus on Kennedy's comments about her prior supervision, deciding in the moment not to give space and time for that topic at this stage. Pin Xiu hoped that by focusing on the future, Kennedy may be able to move on from the negative narrative she had expressed. Pin Xiu also wondered if Kennedy's 'arrogance' was her way of trying to impress the team, or perhaps might be saying something she desperately wanted to believe to cover up insecurities she felt.

In the illustrative example, we can see that Pin Xiu holds the balance of power as the 'captain of the ship', or in the front seat of the Tandem Model of Clinical Supervision (Milne and James, 2005). She attempted to gently steer the discussion to where she thought it would be most useful. This can be an effective supervisory strategy, but it should be used intentionally and with critical self-reflection. This is to ensure we, as supervisors, are not steering the conversation to a place more comfortable for ourselves, or to a place that is unhelpful for both supervisor and supervisee. We pick up the second part of the illustrative example and see how Pin Xiu steers the conversation to focus on how Kennedy could feel more part of the team (**Box 8.12**).

BOX 8.12

Illustrative example: Pin Xiu and Kennedy – changing the narrative

Pin Xiu began by discussing times when Kennedy had felt a part of a team. Kennedy described a range of scenarios that were all situations when Kennedy was with her peers. This was the first time she had worked in a team of people of mixed ages. With her peers, Kennedy felt comfortable with modes of communication, cultural references, in-jokes and felt she could match others' knowledge and skills. Pin Xiu and Kennedy discussed the strengths and capabilities that enabled Kennedy to have such positive team experiences with her peers – good communication, an interest in others, a sense of humour, and a desire to be part of a team.

Kennedy then confided that she had been feeling despondent about working in the organisation. She felt no one liked her and she did not feel confident about her skills, as everyone else in the team was so much older and more experienced. Kennedy considered her behaviour and wondered if, in her attempt to hide her insecurities, she had been 'coming on too strong' in terms of how knowledgeable she had been acting.

Pin Xiu and Kennedy discussed Kennedy's strengths and focused on how she could use the successful communication strategies she has with her peers and transfer them into this situation in an intentional way. Together they came up with a plan to 'tone down' her communication about what she knew and instead amplify her skills in connecting with others, being interested in their lives, appropriately using humour and to ask for help and seek others' opinions more frequently.

Kennedy tried out this approach over the next month, and when she next met with Pin Xiu, reported that people were more friendly with her, engaging in conversations about non-work topics (like the latest television series), and offering and requesting opinions and help on work matters. After three months, Pin Xiu was receiving unsolicited positive comments from team members about how much Kennedy had developed recently.

A question that you may be thinking is, why not just directly confront Kennedy about her behaviour? This is a strategy that can be used, but direct confrontation risks the relationship, and the supervisee can retreat into a position of resistance, making change much harder to achieve. Cojocaru (2010) found they were able to gain profound changes in difficult situations by using an appreciative approach and focusing on what could be, not what currently is. To help you think about your own situation, we invite you to take some time to reflect on Pin Xiu and Kennedy's story using the prompt questions we introduced earlier in Box 8.5. You may like to add to your previous notes and again raise any points of interest in your own supervision or with a trusted peer.

In the illustrative example, we have focused on a **supervisee** that appears to overestimate their abilities and how that may be worked through in supervision. It is possible that a similar appreciative, strengths-based approach would be useful if the supervisee appears to underestimate their abilities. What could be more challenging to address is where it is the **supervisor who appears to over- or underestimate their abilities**. Due to the power and hierarchy inherent in most supervisory relationships, it will be unlikely that the supervisee will have the same control over supervision. In this case, we hope the supervisor will remain open and reflective of their own skills, seek feedback and their own supervisory support. As a supervisee in this situation, you may gently raise your concerns if you feel it is appropriate, or seek additional advice and guidance outside of the supervisory relationship through the creation of your supervisory portfolio.

As a final point in this section, we want to once again raise the idea of diversity in the workplace. We propose that when people perceive someone as over- or underestimating their abilities, part of it may actually be related to **inclusivity and diversity**. Many of us are familiar with the idea of making '**reasonable adjustments**' to workplace practices to enable all of us to contribute to our potential. What is interesting in our view is how as health professionals we are dedicated to making a difference in people's lives through being aware of diversity and making changes to enable occupational engagement, performance, and participation. However, there is evidence that supervisees experience considerable barriers during their education and when in practice settings in supervision, including responses when disclosing a disability; the outcomes when asking for and receiving reasonable accommodations; and attitudinal barriers from supervisors and colleagues (Lund et al., 2020). While we are highlighting inclusivity and diversity in relation to disability, we think that Singh and Chun's (2010) Queer People of Color Resilience-Based Model of Supervision could be helpful to consider multiple identities or intersectionality (as discussed in Chapter 1).

For now, perhaps we are more familiar with making accommodations with the people accessing our services, such as people joining the workforce or returning to work following illness or injury. For example, an evidence synthesis in 2017 by Padkapayeva and colleagues highlighted twelve modification areas for people with physical disabilities in the workplace. Accommodations for people returning to work with mental health conditions are also being reported, such as following depression (Bastien and Corbière, 2019). **Box 8.13** offers a short summary of some common areas of accommodation. These may also be helpful for supervision, although we would encourage wider reading for more information.

BOX 8.13

Common areas of accommodation in the workplace

- Modifications to rules, policies, or practices, e.g. working from home, allowing guide dogs in the workplace, additional supervision sessions, opportunity for ad hoc communication, adjustments to scheduling of work activities, or job restructuring.
- Removal of architectural, communication, or transportation barriers, e.g. workstation adjustments, use of multiple communication strategies, universally accessible buildings, parking.
- Attitudes of others, e.g. a workplace that promotes positive attitudes and social inclusion, policies that are inclusive, options for mediation, commitment to fair performance evaluations, opportunity for further education.
- Provision of auxiliary aids, e.g. dyslexia-friendly software, organisational aids, hearing loops.

Our thoughts here are about how we can use our professional knowledge, skills, and mindset about inclusivity and diversity and apply them in supervision. Being open to exploring potential reasons behind someone's behaviour, whether it be from a lack of awareness; related to inclusivity, diversity, or disability; a coping mechanism; power and hierarchy; role conflicts; or something else, may offer a productive way forward. With the right scaffolding through your portfolio of supervision you can keep your battery charged so your personal and professional self can function effectively. To conclude this chapter, we invite you to reflect on your own supervisory needs with the questions posed in **Box 8.14**.

BOX 8.14

Reflecting on your own supervisory needs

- Think about your own supervisory and professional/career development needs. How are these going to be met and by whom?
- How can you build your own supervisory team? What formal and informal support would you like to have in your supervisory portfolio?
- In your supervisory portfolio, how will you ensure all parties are clear on their roles, and the specific boundaries of their roles?

CRITICAL COMMENTARY

Are we ignoring challenges and problems?

Using an appreciative, strengths-based approach does not mean that challenges are ignored or are only seen in a positive light. Instead, situations are acknowledged for what they are, but there is a belief that a way forward can be found. In writing this chapter, we have debated how far we go down the 'appreciative road'. While we advocate for seeing things in a positive light, we know that we often only pay close attention to things when we see them as a 'problem'. Therefore, we've talked about tensions in supervision because we thought that would be recognisable to many, and then offered a strengths-based and appreciative way to work through those tensions.

When considering the evidence, appreciative, strengths-based approaches have been criticised for not being particularly new, original, or different from approaches already widely used (McMillen et al., 2004; Staudt et al., 2001). However, it does appear to be a common contemporary approach in modern-day practice. For example, in working with people with long-term conditions and disability, and in community development, an 'assets-based' approach is widely utilised; focusing on potential rather than what is lacking (Miller et al., 2018; Kretzmann and McKnight, 1993). If we use assets, focus on potential, and see tensions as something that can be worked through with the support of individuals, organisations, and wider systems, over time we can build on the strengths of supervisors and supervisees.

SUMMARY

In this chapter, we have explored three common tensions we can face in supervision. These tensions relate to support versus performance evaluation; power and hierarchy; and when a supervisor or supervisee appears to over- or underestimate their abilities. Using an appreciative, strengths-based approach is a valuable general skill set to address many of the tensions that might arise within a supervisory relationship. While we have focused largely on what individuals can do in supervision, consideration and support are also needed from organisations and systems to mitigate tensions. Therefore, in the next chapter, we will also draw on appreciative, strengths-based approaches as we consider supervision from managerial and strategic perspectives.

REFERENCES

Bastien, M.-F. and Corbière, M. (2019). 'Return-to-work following depression: what work accommodations do employers and human resources directors put in place?', *Journal of Occupational Rehabilitation*, 29(2), pp. 423–432. doi:10.1007/s10926-018-9801-y.

Berg, C.J. (2009) 'A comprehensive framework for conducting client assessments: highlighting strengths, environmental factors and hope', *Journal of Practical Consulting*, 3(2), pp. 9–13. Available at: www.regent.edu/acad/global/publications/jpc/vol3iss2/JPC_V3Is2_Berg.pdf (Accessed: 16 November 2021).

Brown, O., Kangovi, S., Wiggins, N., and Alvarado, C.S. (2020) *Supervision strategies and community health worker effectiveness in health care settings*. Available at: https://nam.edu/supervision-strategies-and-community-health-worker-effectiveness-in-health-care-settings/ (Accessed: 16 November 2021).

Carlson, D., Ferguson, M., Hunter, E., and Whitten, D. (2012) 'Abusive supervision and work–family conflict: the path through emotional labor and burnout', *The Leadership Quarterly*, 23(5), pp. 849–859. doi:10.1016/j.leaqua.2012.05.003.

Cojocaru, S. (2010) 'Appreciative supervision in social work: new opportunities for changing the social work practice', *Revista de Cercetare şi Intervenţie Socială*, 29, pp. 72–91.

Cooperrider, D. (2013) 'A contemporary commentary on *Appreciative Inquiry in Organizational Life*', in Cooperrider, D., Zandee, D., Godwin, L., Avital, M., and Boland, B. (eds) *Organizational Generativity: The Appreciative Inquiry Summit and a Scholarship of Transformation*. Bingley: Emerald Publishing, pp. 3–67. doi:10.1108/S1475-9152(2013)0000004001.

Cooperrider, D. and Srivastva, S. (1987). 'Appreciative inquiry in organizational life'. In Woodman, R. and Pasmore, W. (eds) *Research in organizational change and development*, vol. 1. Bingley: Emerald Publishing, pp. 129–169.

Cooperrider, D., Whitney, D.D., and Stavros, J., (2008) *The appreciative inquiry handbook: for leaders of change*. Oakland, CA: Berrett-Koehler Publishers.

Davys, A. and Beddoe, L., 2020. *Best practice in professional supervision: a guide for the helping professions*. London: Jessica Kingsley Publishers.

Falender, C.A. (2009) 'Relationship and accountability: tensions in feminist supervision', *Women and Therapy*, 33(1–2), pp. 22–41. doi:10.1080/02703140903404697.

Fialkov, C. and Haddad, D. (2012) 'Appreciative clinical training', *Training and Education in Professional Psychology*, 6(4), pp. 204–210. doi:10.1037/a0030832.

González, R. C. (1997) 'Postmodern supervision', *Multicultural Counseling Competencies: Assessment, Education and Training, and Supervision*, 7, pp. 350–386.

Graybeal, C. (2001) 'Strengths-based social work assessment: transforming the dominant paradigm', *Families in Society*, 82(3), pp. 233–242. doi:10.1606/1044-3894.236.

Kretzmann, J.P. and McKnight, J.L. (1993) Asset-based community development: mobilizing an entire community, in Kretzmann, J.P. and McKnight, J.L. (eds) *Building Communities from the Inside Out: A Path towards Finding and Mobilizing a Community's Assets*. Chicago, IL: ACTA Publications, pp. 345–354.

Luft, J. and Ingham, H. (1955) 'The Johari window, a graphic model of interpersonal awareness', *Proceedings of the Western Training Laboratory in Group Development*. Los Angeles, CA: UCLA.

Lund, E.M., Wilbur, R.C., and Kuemmel, A.M. (2020) 'Beyond legal obligation: the role and necessity of the supervisor-advocate in creating a socially just, disability-affirmative training environment', *Training and Education in Professional Psychology*, 14(2) pp. 92–99. doi:10.1037/tep0000277.

Masters, M.A. (1992) 'The use of positive reframing in the context of supervision', *Journal of Counseling and Development*, 70(3), pp. 387–390. doi:10.1002/j.1556-6676.1992.tb01621.x.

McMillen, J.C., Morris, L., and Sherraden, M. (2004) 'Ending social work's grudge match: problems versus strengths', *Families in Society*, 85(3), pp. 317–325. doi:10.1177/104438940408500309.

Mette, I.M., Range, B.G., Anderson, J., Hvidston, D.J., Nieuwenhuizen, L., and Doty, J. (2017) 'The wicked problem of the intersection between supervision and evaluation', *International Electronic Journal of Elementary Education*, 9(3), pp. 709–724. Available at: www.iejee.com/index.php/IEJEE/article/view/185 (Accessed: 16 November 2021).

Miller, K., McIntyre, R., and McKenna, G. (2018) 'Assets based community participation and place making', *Journal of Finnish Universities of Applied Sciences*, 4. Available at: https://uasjournal.fi/in-english/assets-based-community-participation/ (Accessed: 16 November 2021).

Milne, D. and James, I. (2005) 'Clinical supervision: ten tests of the tandem model', *Clinical Psychology Forum*, 151, pp. 6–10.

Padkapayeva, K., Posen, A., Yazdani, A. Buettgen, A., Mahood, Q., and Tompa, E. (2017) 'Workplace accommodations for persons with physical disabilities: evidence synthesis of the peer-reviewed literature', *Disability and Rehabilitation*, 39(21), pp. 2134–2147. doi:10.1080/09638288.2016.1224276.

Rapp, C., Saleebey, D., and Sullivan, P.W. (2008) 'The future of strengths-based social work practice 2006', in Saleebey, D. (ed.) *The strengths perspective in social work practice*. 4th edn. Boston: Pearson Education.

Ryde, J. (2009) *Being white in the helping professions: developing effective intercultural awareness.* London: Jessica Kingsley Publishers.

Schreibman, R. and Chilton, G. (2012) 'Small waterfalls in art therapy supervision: a poetic appreciative inquiry', *Art Therapy*, 29(4), pp. 188–191. doi:10.1080/07421656.2012.730924.

Singh, A. and Chun, K.Y.S. (2010) '"From the margins to the center": moving towards a resilience-based model of supervision for queer people of color supervisors', *Training and Education in Professional Psychology*, 4(1), pp. 36–46. doi:10.1037/a0017373.

Staudt, M., Howard, M.O., and Drake, B. (2001) 'The operationalization, implementation, and effectiveness of the strengths perspective: a review of empirical studies', *Journal of Social Service Research*, 27(3), pp. 1–21. doi:10.1300/J079v27n03_01.

Stavros, J., Torres, C.B., and Cooperrider, D.L. (2018) *Conversations worth having: using appreciative inquiry to fuel productive and meaningful engagement.* Oakland, CA: Berrett-Koehler Publishers.

Tsui, M.-S. (2004). 'Supervision models in social work: From nature to culture', *Asian Journal of Counselling*, 11(1–2), pp. 7–55.

Wang, E.A., Riley, C., Wood, G., Greene, A., Horton, N., Williams, M., Violano, P., Brase, R.M., Brinkley-Rubinstein, L., Papachristos, A.V., and Roy, B. (2020) 'Building community resilience to prevent and mitigate community impact of gun violence: conceptual framework and intervention design', *BMJ Open*, 10(10), article e040277, pp. 1–8.

Wong, S.R., Ngooi, B.X., Kwa, F.Y., Koh, X.T., Chua, R.J., and Dancza, K. (2021). 'Exploring the meaning of value-based occupational therapy services from the perspectives of managers, therapists and clients', *British Journal of Occupational Therapy.* doi:10.1177/03080226211030095.

Appendix 8.1: Strengths-Based Self-Evaluation Tool for Supervisors guidance template (adapted from Rapp et al., 2008)

As a supervisor, am I goal-focused?	
• Are goals a feature of my supervision? • Do I facilitate my supervisee(s) to set their own goals for what they want to achieve from supervision?	Notes:

As a supervisor, am I maximising available resources?	
• Have I considered who or what information or resources exist that may help the supervisee(s)? • Do I encourage my supervisee(s) to identify available resources and plan how to access them?	Notes:

As a supervisor, am I making strengths explicit?	
• Do I know what strengths my supervisee(s) have? • Do I encourage acknowledgement of strengths?	Notes:

As a supervisor, am I expressing hope?	
• Do I have a positive outlook in supervision sessions? • Do I express hopefulness when interacting with my supervisee(s)?	Notes:

As a supervisor, am I offering meaningful choice?	
• Do I see my supervisee(s) as able to make decisions? • Have I supported people making informed choices?	**Notes:**
As a supervisor, am I strengths-focused?	
• Do I identify and draw on capabilities of the supervisee(s)? • Do I acknowledge challenges and support the supervisee(s) to find ways to change or adapt to the situation?	**Notes:**

Appendix 8.2: Reflection activity using the Johari Window (adapted from Luft and Ingham, 1955)

1. Create your own Johari Window

• Think about situations you have experienced recently in your work. Make a list of your qualities, knowledge, and skills that may be positive or things you are less confident with.
• Draw your own Johari Window. Map your list of qualities, knowledge, and skills into either:
  o **Open self** – for things you are happy to share with others
  o **Hidden self** – for things you prefer to keep to yourself (perhaps a lack of confidence or quality you are not so proud of).

2. Gaining feedback from a trusted person
• Sharing your window with someone you trust (as honestly as you feel comfortable with), enables them to help you see your blind self. Ask this trusted person if they can add any information about your qualities, knowledge, and skills into the blind self-window. • If you don't have someone you want to share your window with, imagine you are someone that you look up to / a person who accesses your services / a former mentor – what might they say about you? What other qualities, knowledge, and skills might they add to your blind self-window?
3. Did you learn anything new?
• From your feedback (real or imagined), did anything in your window change? • Were you able to move anything from your hidden self to your open self? Or move something from your blind self to your open or hidden self? • Did your reflections make you consider some things in your unknown self-window? • This activity is intended as a starting point for discussions. You may like to consider other reflective tools or techniques and perhaps return to your window after some time and see if anything has changed.

CHAPTER 9

Effective supervision from managerial and strategic perspectives

Cate Fitzgerald, Christine Craik, Stephanie Tempest, and Karina Dancza

With contributions from Helen Hak, Samreen Jawaid, Maha Sohail, Margaret Spencer, Anita Volkert, and Debbie Kramer-Roy

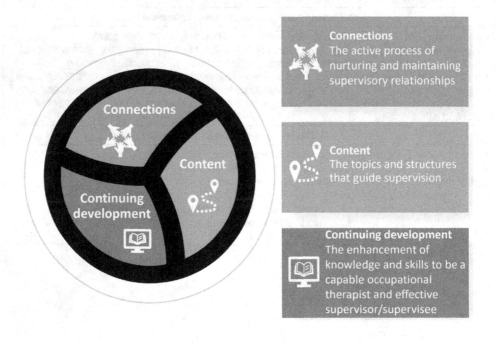

Connections
The active process of nurturing and maintaining supervisory relationships

Content
The topics and structures that guide supervision

Continuing development
The enhancement of knowledge and skills to be a capable occupational therapist and effective supervisor/supervisee

DOI: 10.4324/9781003092544-9

CHAPTER INTENTIONS

In this chapter we invite you to:

- Explore the content of supervision from an organisational perspective
- Consider ways to enhance the quality of supervision at department, organisational, and system levels
- Identify strategic ways to enhance connection and inclusive supervisory practices in the workplace
- Review continuing development needs from a whole service perspective
- Examine different ways to measure the impact of supervision.

CHAPTER HIGHLIGHTS

- Supervision from managerial and strategic perspectives
- Content and ensuring quality in supervision systems
- Connections and enhancing inclusive supervision in the workplace
- Continuing development of supervisees, supervisors, and managers
- Measuring the impact of supervision
- Critical commentary: The value placed on supervision

CHAPTER RESOURCES

Figure

- Figure 9.1 General steps of creating a business case

Tables

- Table 9.1 Priorities for the content of supervision according to organisational governance and supervisees' needs
- Table 9.2 Examples of tools to measure supervision

Boxes

- Box 9.1 Resources to build a case for change to organisational supervisory practices
- Box 9.2 Reflective Story by Helen Hak: Evaluating supervision processes in a large organisation
- Box 9.3 Reflective Story by Helen Hak: Acknowledging the tensions in the functions of supervision

- Box 9.4 Ideas to help navigate being a supervisor and line manager
- Box 9.5 Editor's Reflective Story: Developing a business case
- Box 9.6 Three top tips for developing a business case
- Box 9.7 Workplace changes to create a positive and affirming supervision culture
- Box 9.8 Reflective Story by Helen Hak: Establishing trust in supervision
- Box 9.9 Questions to consider at managerial and strategic levels to develop inclusive supervision
- Box 9.10 Reflective Story by Samreen Jawaid and Maha Sohail: Using action research to develop supervision
- Box 9.11 Ideas for when the supervisee's and manager's professional development priorities differ
- Box 9.12 Reflective Story by Margaret Spencer: Diverse practice-based learning and supervision to develop new services
- Box 9.13 Measuring effective supervision – what exactly are we measuring?

SUPERVISION FROM MANAGERIAL AND STRATEGIC PERSPECTIVES

Supervision serves as a mechanism for public and professional safety. For this reason, along with a range of other benefits, supervision is an asset to managers of services and strategic leaders (Rice et al., 2020). For example, high-quality supervision has been associated with improved staff wellbeing (Winstanley and White, 2003); staff perception of better patient outcomes (Busari and Koot, 2007); supports staff to maintain competence and enhances their practice (Strong et al, 2003); and can positively impact on staff retention (Dancza et al., 2021). It is no surprise then that supervision is often incorporated into professional governance systems within organisations (Martin et al., 2017). But there is still work to do.

In this chapter we will explore supervision from the perspectives of middle managers, those who work at an operational level within a team, service, or department, and senior managers and leaders who are responsible for the strategic direction of the organisation. We will use the 3Cs for Effective Supervision – **Connections, Content, Continuing development** – to frame the operational and strategic management aspects within occupational therapy supervision. To begin we will consider the **Content** of supervision.

CONTENT AND ENSURING QUALITY IN SUPERVISION SYSTEMS

When supervision is embedded in the broader workplace culture, there will be structures, policies, and systems in place to support its effective implementation. As a manager, being familiar with these policies and procedures, and understanding the skills of your supervisors and supervisees in your team, will enable you to make the most of the talent you have. A key role of a manager is to **create supervisory practices that are meaningful for your team and aligned with organisational systems**. This can be a delicate balance that requires a critical eye on the needs of the team and the organisational systems, in part so you can influence the future evolution of supervisory practice and policies when they are reviewed.

When comprehensive supervision structures such as policies, guidelines, and resources are not available or lack sufficient detail, this poses a risk to the quality of supervision and therefore the delivery of safe and effective services. Therefore, managers and strategic leaders may be involved in developing a supervisory strategy at a team, department, or whole service level. We invite you to consider some resources and guidance that can help build a case for enhancements to supervisory practices in **Box 9.1**.

BOX 9.1

Resources to build a case for change to organisational supervisory practices

- Occupational therapy professional associations can offer scope of practice, ethical, and supervisory frameworks that advocate the need for supervision. For example, Occupational Therapy Australia (OTA)'s Occupational Therapy Scope of Practice Framework states that occupational therapists have a responsibility "to ensure currency of practice, registration, and contemporary professional knowledge by seeking appropriate professional supervision, training and professional development to maintain practice within the scope of practice" (OTA, 2017, p. 6, cited in OTA, 2019). OTA have also developed national guidance for supervision (OTA, 2019).
- Professional registration boards and healthcare systems regulators may also offer professional supervision frameworks with recommendations for professional development. For example, the Health and Care Professions Council (HCPC) in the United Kingdom provides several online resources e.g. a webinar on delegation, research on effective supervision characteristics (see Chapter 1; HCPC, 2020), and standards for supervision.
- Governing authority of the broader health and care system may also offer guidance that is not always profession specific. These resources can help you create a case for supervision and articulate the minimum standards by which supervision practices can be evaluated.
- Supervisory frameworks may be particularly valuable where policies, structures, and guides for the provision of supervision are limited. For example, the 13 domains of supervision outlined in Nancarrow et al. (2014) provide common broad principles that could be applied to local contexts (as outlined in Chapter 1) alongside the overarching use of the 3Cs for Effective Supervision to frame a supervision strategy.

Introducing a change in practice can be challenging, and having the policies, structures, and guidance documents is only part of the story. Next steps often include how to embed changes to the practices of supervision into workplace professional education, support, and administrative functions. We will explore a framework to guide changes to supervisory practices when we discuss learning from implementation science in Chapter 10, but now we would like to invite you to read a **Reflective Story** by Helen Hak (**Box 9.2**). Helen is a strategic clinical lead occupational therapist in the United Kingdom, and she shares how in 2020 she evaluated the perceptions of the supervision processes in her service. Helen was able to create change in supervisory practices by using the evidence generated from her research.

BOX 9.2

Reflective Story by Helen Hak: Evaluating supervision processes in a large organisation

As a strategic clinical lead for occupational therapy in the United Kingdom, I decided to conduct a service evaluation as part of my master's of advanced practice studies in 2019/2020. I am fortunate to work in a service that values supervision and has embedded structures in place. I used the National Health Service Evaluation Cycle (Evaluation Works, n.d.) to evaluate the supervision that occupational therapists received. I interviewed the heads of service of the five specialities: adult physical, mental health, paediatrics, learning disabilities, and complex care. In addition, the 157 registered occupational therapists in the service were invited to complete an electronic questionnaire. I received 71 completed questionnaires (45% response rate) and considered that this offered a reasonable representation of the views of therapists at that time.

Overall, most occupational therapists had positive experiences of supervision and found the current framework and structures supported them. Almost a third of the 71 therapists included the word 'structure' when giving their definition of supervision with one noting that "The overall structure within the service helps, that emphasis is placed on regular supervision ... so that it is prioritised." They felt that supervision fostered the development of themselves as occupational therapists and ensured quality and governance in relation to their practice. However, definitions provided by respondents indicated they felt less emphasis was placed on the wellbeing aspect of supervision.

We will return to Helen's experience throughout this chapter to illustrate our discussions. At this stage, the point we would like to focus on is that, in Helen's service, the embedded supervision structure was valued by the occupational therapists. Creating this structure can, however, become complicated when it needs to address different priorities simultaneously. Broadly speaking, we can think about two main parties, the organisation and the supervisee. We have suggested some of the potential priorities each may have for supervision in **Table 9.1**.

TABLE 9.1 Priorities for the content of supervision according to organisational governance and supervisees' needs

Organisational governance priorities for supervision	Supervisees' priorities for supervision
• Ensuring that people receive safe and effective services • Ensuring that people who access the services are experiencing quality and value • Ensuring occupational therapists work effectively and adapt quickly to evolving environments and expectations of professional performance • Ensuring occupational therapists practise within their role boundaries, professional scope, and aligning these with the organisation's goals for service provision	• To support my continued development • To support me to maintain my own health and wellbeing • To provide a safe space to share my concerns, work through issues, and enhance my learning and practice • To help me navigate workplace complexities successfully

The content of supervision needs to balance organisational governance priorities with the supervisee's priorities. And while there is overlap, this is often where a tension lies. When supervision is viewed as a mechanism to support organisational governance, it is also typically embedded within employee performance management and appraisal systems. But when people feel constantly under scrutiny e.g. when normative functions dominate the restorative (supportive) and formative (educative) functions of supervision (Proctor, 2001), supervisees may not wish to be open about their performance. This tension was illustrated in Helen's study findings (**Box 9.3**).

BOX 9.3

Reflective Story by Helen Hak: Acknowledging the tensions in the functions of supervision

The occupational therapists in my study defined what supervision meant to them. In doing this, their responses strongly reflected two main areas. First, respondents felt strongly that supervision was to support their clinical practice, and this appeared in 56 of the 71 definitions of supervision provided. Second, respondents were also clear that they felt supervision was a tool to enhance quality and governance, with this aspect appearing in 39 definitions. This aligns with other results, with 90% of supervisees reporting confidence that their supervision would address any difficulties or concerns with their practice and all lead therapists expressing confidence that supervision in their teams would address quality and governance issues.

The survey also revealed that 91% of the 71 therapists received supervision from an occupational therapist who was their direct senior or line manager. A concern was raised about potentially conflicting supervisory priorities, as one respondent shared, "You can't always be completely honest if there is a line management structure in place". While the dual role of supervisor and line manager was a satisfactory arrangement for most people, some reported a negative experience leading to the normative, formative, and restorative functions not being balanced appropriately to meet their needs.

Some services, organisations, and professional bodies recommend, where possible, that line management and supervision responsibilities are kept separate to minimise the tensions caused by the duality of the roles. Using a framework embedded into supervision and the policies that support it, offers a potential way to navigate through the tensions by offering a structure which allows recognition for both organisational and professional development. Building on our introduction of Proctor's three functions of supervision in Chapter 1 (Proctor, 2001), in this next section we will reflect on each function (formative, restorative, and normative) from the perspective of managers and strategic leaders.

Formative or educational function of supervision

Within the educational function of supervision, managers and leaders in occupational therapy concentrate on how supervision contributes to the growth of knowledge and skills of people they are responsible for in the organisation. As a manager or leader, we invite you to reflect on how supervision assists therapists to bring evidence into practice, how it stimulates a passion for research in practice, the translation of research outcomes to practice, and how it contributes to developing and consolidating new knowledge and skills required by the organisation.

Restorative or supportive function of supervision

The supportive function of supervision aims to contribute to the professional and personal growth of occupational therapists to sustain their professional practice and own wellbeing. There are many benefits to the organisation and to the people who access services when therapists feel valued and included. For managers and leaders, we invite you to reflect on how supervision encourages supervisees to reflect safely and ethically on their professional scope of practice, identify areas for their learning and development, consider their desires for career advancement, and establish their identity and sense of belonging within an interprofessional team.

Normative or managerial/administrative function of supervision

Supervision serves a protective function for the organisation and the people who access its services through monitoring the adherence to relevant policies, procedures, guidelines, etc. associated with the therapists' role. For managers and leaders, we invite you to reflect on how the administrative function of supervision aims to ensure public and professional safety, and the quality of care.

As previously mentioned, some organisations separate the managerial/administrative function of supervision (line management) from the educative and supportive functions by engaging different supervisors. In others, like Helen described, one supervisor holds both roles. Tension can be caused by the duality of roles, and while there are many ways to approach this, we have offered a few ideas in **Box 9.4**.

BOX 9.4

Ideas to help navigate being a supervisor and line manager

- The use of a supervision model, e.g. Proctor's three functions of supervision (Proctor, 2001), can help to articulate the interactivity of the managerial, educative, and supportive aspects of supervision. Reflecting on the contribution of each aspect to supervision sessions can support a balanced approach.
- Aim for transparency and being open about what is being addressed in supervision (see Chapter 8). Take time to discuss and inform your team about how supervision will be linked, or not, to line management and performance appraisal. This could also form part of a supervision arrangement (see Chapter 5).
- Take extra time to form the connections with yourself and with your supervisee (see chapters 1 and 4).
- Consider if more than one supervisor is needed to achieve and balance the requirements of the organisation and the occupational therapist. If so, it may be possible to create a business case or consider different ways that supervision can be delivered (e.g. group supervision, see Chapter 7).

One of the ideas presented in Box 9.4 suggests creating a business case to support building supervision structures within an organisation or team. In the **Editor's Reflective Story** by Anita, she shares her experiences of building a business case, something that may be familiar to experienced managers **(Box 9.5)**. Some universities include innovation and business elements in their occupational therapy programmes, which is excellent preparation for the current and future work environments, but it is not universal, and revisiting ideas once in a work situation can be helpful. For now, let's hear from Anita and her experience developing a business case.

BOX 9.5

Editor's Reflective Story: Developing a business case

In my own career, I (Anita) first needed to build a business case about five years into my career when I was a senior occupational therapist. I was working within the public health sector, and additional money was available via a charity to potentially fund a specialist oncology occupational therapist. All we needed to do was write a business case to the charity, and formally present our proposal. While I knew what the role for occupational therapy was in the setting, and I had the support of the head of the department (who was also my supervisor), neither of us had created a business case before.

So, we applied the occupational therapy process to the situation. **Step 1** was to gather information about what others had done, seeking out people with similar experiences, finding examples and templates that would help. **Step 2** was to create our timeline, which in this case was only a few weeks. **Step 3** was to outline our expected outcomes (completed business case and presentation) and allocate work tasks. My role was to prepare the first draft of the proposal and presentation, and we refined it together. **Step 4** was to seek feedback from peers and colleagues on our proposal prior to the formal submission and presentation.

Our business case was successful, and we were granted one full-time senior therapist and one part-time entry-level therapist for an initial two-year period, which exceeded our expectations.

To develop a successful business case, we had to 'think differently'. Instead of thinking only about the benefit to those who accessed our services, we had to think economically as well – what were the economic, as well as the health and wellbeing benefits of having these additional therapists in post? How would we know they were making difference? How could we demonstrate that to the funder (the charity) at interim points in the two-year period?

Our learning from the business case and presentation was a key moment in my own career. The need to focus on outcomes led me to include much more rigorous outcome measurements in my work, which was the springboard to some significant career choices later on.

Being a manager or strategic leader can be a steep learning curve. If you are new to leadership or management, or indeed at any career stage, you may like to consider your own supervision, mentoring or coaching and how it supports your role. The appropriate support for you may come from someone outside of our profession with a business or managerial background.

There are many useful examples of business case templates online and we would encourage anyone who is unfamiliar with this process to explore these for ideas. As a general approach to creating a business case, we have shared a three-step process by Think Pacific (2020) in **Figure 9.1**.

Whether you are developing a business case for a new service, member of staff, supervision development, or anything else, we would like to share our three top tips in **Box 9.6**

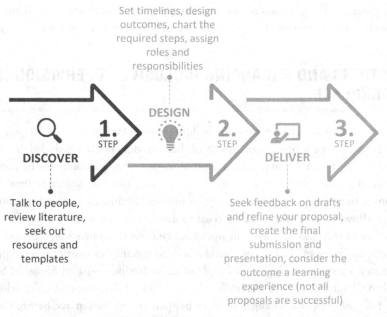

FIGURE 9.1 General steps of creating a business case (adapted from Think Pacific, 2020)

BOX 9.6

Three top tips for developing a business case

- You may find yourself out of your comfort zone but embrace the learning and development opportunity – you may get better results than you imagine.
- Use your own supervision; if you are a supervisor and this is new for you too, learn with your supervisee.
- Use your wider networks (both supervisor and supervisee) for ideas and feedback on initial drafts. Try to share your ideas along the way so you remain open and accepting of feedback, rather than asking for feedback when the deadlines are too close for you to change your proposal.

Ultimately, managers or leaders with supervision and management responsibilities need to be aware of governance and the duty of care to people who access services and the organisation, especially as you take on roles and responsibilities which require the escalation of unsafe practice. From a managerial and strategic perspective, there will always be a need to view supervision as operating within the organisational requirements for performance management.

Keeping this focus, it will need to be balanced with meeting the supervisees' educative and supportive needs, requiring a sometimes-delicate balancing act. Recognising the different content priorities and allocating or generating resources to address them is an important strategy, but it is enhanced by having strong **Connections** within supervisory relationships and demonstrating a culture of inclusivity in the workplace. This will be explored in the next section.

CONNECTIONS AND ENHANCING INCLUSIVE SUPERVISION IN THE WORKPLACE

Central to the supervisory relationship is the building of trust (as discussed in Chapter 4). Yet this is a challenge when, for example, an occupational therapist does not feel included or valued in the workplace culture. This could happen for a range of reasons. One possibility is when occupational therapists are in a rotational position in the team, they may not have sufficient time to establish Connections if they change supervisors every six months. Strategic consideration can make the difference in **allowing time and space for trust to develop** (as discussed in Chapter 1).

Other factors may also be present in workplace cultures that impact on a person's feeling of being valued and included. To help us consider how to enhance inclusivity in workplace supervision practices, we return to the Queer People of Color Resilience-Based Model of Supervision introduced in Chapter 1. In their model, Singh and Chun (2010) emphasise the value of inclusivity, and take the view that **changes need to happen in the workplace before the purpose of supervision to support supervisee development can be fully realised**. For these workplace changes to be truly effective, it requires managerial and organisational level support. Some examples of workplace changes are shared in **Box 9.7**.

BOX 9.7

Workplace changes to create a positive and affirming supervision culture (adapted from Singh and Chun, 2010)

- An attitude of inclusivity reflected throughout the workplace. For example, recruitment processes that welcome diversity, and symbols and signs of diversity and inclusivity within materials and decor.
- A lifelong commitment to quality learning opportunities on cultural humility and diversity for all employees, including supervisees and supervisors.
- At the beginning of supervisory relationships, supervisors can explore ways in which multiple identities (intersectionality) may influence supervisees' conceptualisation of the people who access the services, and their histories of resilience and oppression.
- To not rely on a few 'diverse' people to have to 'educate' all other employees about issues of diversity and how to respond.

How people experience workplace cultures will also be diverse. When exploring how to enhance people's feelings of being included and valued in an organisation, it is important to actively **understand current and past supervision experiences**, including the positive or negative impact on the motivation for people to engage in supervision, as both a supervisor and a supervisee. This need is highlighted in our next instalment of Helen's **Reflective Story**, where she reports that while most therapists had positive experiences, some therapists were not satisfied with their current supervisory arrangements **(Box 9.8)**. This feedback was then used by managers to drive improvements to the supervisory provision within their service.

BOX 9.8

Reflective Story by Helen Hak: Establishing trust in supervision

In my service evaluation, most occupational therapists reported a positive experience of supervision, and 88% of the 71 occupational therapists were positive about how trustworthy they felt their supervisory relationship was.

When asked to rate if their supervision had met their expectations, 21% of respondents provided a negative score. Narrative responses suggested that hierarchical allocation of supervisors could be a contributing factor for those experiencing challenges. One noted "it is very hard for someone to go over their supervisor's head to discuss with a higher manager". Other comments reflected dissatisfaction linked to problems with trust within the supervisory relationship. One occupational therapist said, "I often feel inadequate and like I am being scrutinised", and another "my current supervision is really unhelpful, it reduces my confidence and is not a safe place to discuss anything".

Positively, even though supervision did not always meet expectations, 97% of respondents felt able to expose weaknesses and mistakes within supervision. As a service we were aware of the need to prioritise the development of positive, trusting supervisory relationships particularly for those therapists who reported concerns or issues. It was clear from the service evaluation that the relationship between supervisor and supervisee was central to effective supervision. Established processes and expectations within our service meant we could begin to look at these more complex aspects of supervision.

When someone has experienced less-than-optimal supervision, they may develop negative perspectives, unhelpful habits, or supervision practices that create barriers to them gaining the full benefits of supervision. The same could be said for supervisors. It is also possible that, over time, people develop tolerance of poor supervision practices. When this occurs, it is challenging for managers and the organisation to motivate engagement in supervision.

When faced with these types of challenges, it may be helpful to return to the concept of inclusive supervision and consider some of the strategies that can promote Connections from the perspective of managerial and strategic levels. **Box 9.9** offers exploratory questions for considering inclusive supervision based on the Identity-Conscious Supervision Model (Brown et al., 2019). As you read the questions, think about what you already know about your organisational policies, the learning and development opportunities available to you, and how you might access funding for specific educational needs. It can also be helpful to identify what is within your control that can influence and activate change.

BOX 9.9

Questions to consider at managerial and strategic levels to develop inclusive supervision (adapted from Brown et al., 2019)

Relationship with self and others

- How does the organisation support the development of safe supervisory spaces?
- What systems are in place to enable supervisees and supervisors to develop and maintain effective connections?
- Is there protected time for supervision activities?

Creating a strong sense of self

- What opportunities are available for supervisors to develop their intrapersonal knowledge and skills, to acknowledge and address their own biases, knowledge gaps, sources of discomfort, etc.?
- Are there any general courses offered within the human resource function that provide transferable knowledge and skills to aid the development of inclusive supervision?
- Is there access to coaching and/or counselling services in the event supervisors need support with their own self-work, including to understand and process the impact of their dominant and marginalised identities on their ability to be an effective supervisor?

Managing power

- What is available to supervisors and supervisees to enable them to effectively manage the power dynamics that are inherent within the supervisory process? For example, is there an opportunity for 360-degree feedback within the appraisal system?

Acting with courage

- What support and systems are in place to help supervisors and supervisees act with courage and raise issues e.g. about the institutional or departmental supervision culture?
- How does the organisation learn from mistakes and how is this represented through broader policies e.g. whistleblowing policies?
- How is the impact of change measured at organisational and strategic levels?

Fostering identity exploration

- Is there a clear role or job description for a supervisor and supervisee within your organisation?
- Is it clear who will do what and the responsibilities each person has within the relationship?
- Is there a supervision arrangement, agreement, or contract?
- Is the supervision arrangement inclusive and contemporary to meet the evolving needs of the multi-generational workforce?

Balancing expectations and identity

- Is supervision identified as an expected task within broader job descriptions? If so, is there clarity on the differences between formative, normative, and restorative functions of supervision (Proctor, 2001)?
- Does the broader organisation identify who is responsible for the strategic development of supervision?
- Is there a policy that places supervision within the context of continuing professional development?
- Do supervisory policies reflect supervision as a public and professional safety mechanism? Are links made between supervision and the effectiveness of services for people who access them?

Engaging with conflict

- How are employees supported to develop skills in managing and resolving conflict?
- What systems and supportive functions exist to mediate if support is required to resolve conflict between the supervisor and supervisee?

Sustaining identity-consciousness

- What support is in place to help supervisors and supervisees apply their knowledge of inclusive supervision/identity consciousness into practice?
- Are there regular opportunities to review progress in the iterative development to become an inclusive supervisor/supervisee?

Influencing institutional change

- How can supervisors and supervisees be supported to identify what is within their sphere of influence, with the intent to change the culture of supervisory practices within the organisation?
- What alliances/networks exist or can be created within the organisation to build the momentum for quality improvements in supervisory practices?
- Who is there within the system at a range of levels who can help identify the broader 'pain points' in the organisation? How can changes in supervisory practices help to soothe these pain points?
- What organisational values exist in the system that either help or hinder the development of supervisory practices?

As you consider these questions, you may find there are gaps within the structures, policies, and opportunities available within your service and organisation. In our next **Reflective Story** by Samreen Jawaid (teacher) and Maha Sohail (occupational therapist), they illustrate how they used an action research project to create their own supervision opportunities and structures as they worked together in a school in Pakistan (**Box 9.10**; Kramer-Roy et al., 2020).

BOX 9.10

Reflective Story by Samreen Jawaid and Maha Sohail: Using action research to develop supervision

During our action research project, occupational therapists and teachers worked together in different schools to promote inclusive education. This was a unique experience because, in Pakistan, opportunities for inter-professional working are rare. Discovering how we could work together effectively as occupational therapists and teachers was crucial and enhanced our professional development. Here are some of our reflections of the experience.

Samreen: As a teacher, before the action research project, I looked for information on the internet and attended occasional training sessions for help on how to include children in my class with disabilities such as autism. It wasn't until Maha (who is an occupational therapist) and I carried out classroom observations together that we were able to comprehensively identify why a child was experiencing challenges in my class.

Maha's knowledge and experience helped me understand why a child was unable to follow instructions and communicate with his peers and me. By reflecting and sharing strategies we developed an effective inclusive plan for this child, focusing on the classroom environment and the tasks and activities offered in the class. Coming from two different professional backgrounds we were able to see things from new perspectives and draw on each of our strengths to help this child, and others, participate in class.

Maha: Working together helped me as an occupational therapist to gain an understanding of the struggles children with special needs face when participating in the classroom. I learned how teachers worked with the children and started appreciating the complex and strenuous task of teaching a large mainstream class with several children with different special needs.

Even though it was initially hard for us to accept and understand each other's way of perceiving the situation, the structured approach of our action research project, including the use of joint reflective logs, made us into a strong team. By using supervision within the research process, we were able to come up with the strategies together, the teachers were able to make them realistic and they were motivated to implement them consistently.

Samreen and Maha highlighted how supervisory opportunities may come from unexpected places. As a manager, being open and supportive of projects and relationships that are created by team members, with colleagues within and outside the organisation, or through professional associations could offer new avenues for creative supervisory options. In our final C for Effective Supervision, we will focus on ways to support **Continuing development** from managerial and strategic perspectives.

CONTINUING DEVELOPMENT OF SUPERVISEES, SUPERVISORS, AND MANAGERS

It has long been argued that the workplace is dominated by noise and haste, rather than space and silence (Dawson, 2003). This makes it difficult to create time to critically reflect, learn, and develop. As strategic leaders and managers, there is a need to find the balance between the often frantic pace and culture and the opportunities to engage in meaningful supervision and develop new ways of providing supervisory support. We will focus first on the managerial support needs for supervisees' professional development, and then turn our attention to supporting supervisors, managers, and strategic leaders to continue theirs.

Managers' role in the continuing professional development of supervisees

In systems with finite resources, as a manager you will likely need to advocate for, or approve, the supervisees' learning goals and educational options. This approval needs to consider the **cost** (e.g. time out of the workplace or registration cost of the educational activity) and **benefit** of the activity (e.g., meaningfulness, usefulness, and applicability of learning to the person and team). Tension may arise if views of suitable learning goals and educational opportunities differ between supervisee and manager. **Box 9.11** offers a few ideas for how to approach this situation.

BOX 9.11

Ideas for when the supervisee's and manager's professional development priorities differ

- Explore with the supervisee the motivation behind the creation of this learning goal or request for educational opportunity. For example, does the supervisee want to explore a new direction or gain an additional qualification to open future opportunities? Would an investment in the supervisee now help to retain them in the organisation?
- Consider potential areas for negotiation. For example, is there a similar learning opportunity available that is more acceptable to the organisation? Could an opportunity be created for group learning to maximise value for money? Could time be allocated if funds are unavailable?
- Discuss with the supervisee their short-, medium-, and long-term plans to map out current and future opportunities that are meaningful to them and helpful for the organisation. For example, if an early career therapist would like to supervise, can they be involved in student supervision? If a person would like to explore research, can they be mentored or enrolled in a higher degree?

Development opportunities are needed regardless of career stage, and we will now turn our attention to the professional development for supervisors.

Managers' role in the continuing professional development of supervisors

The skills of a supervisor are pivotal in influencing the quality of supervision. Since supervision has been associated with a range of benefits for the organisation and individuals, from a management or strategic viewpoint, it makes sense to focus on developmental support for supervisors. For example, Deci and Ryan (2010) propose that if a supervisor uses authentic praise and positive messaging while providing optimal challenge, then supervisees benefit through enhancing enjoyment and interest in their work and their perception of their own competence in the workplace. A qualitative study involving early career occupational therapists and social workers reported that a positive supervisor and supervisee relationship benefited supervisees through directing their professional career development, supporting them to keep track of their caseload as well as aiding them to identify learning needs (Pack, 2015). Thus, having supervisory skills as a focus in professional development planning is likely to have benefits for both supervisors and supervisees.

The importance of a skilled supervisor is illustrated in the **Reflective Story** by Margaret Spencer (**Box 9.12**). She explains how quality external occupational therapy supervision that began from a student fieldwork placement, enabled the development of a new occupational therapy service. The story highlights how a long-term connection between the external supervisor and supervisee created not only a valued service, but also a new opportunity for the supervisee to become the supervisor as the service was expanded.

BOX 9.12

Reflective Story by Margaret Spencer: Diverse practice-based learning and supervision to develop new services

This story begins as a role emerging placement in a transgender service. The service, although part of the National Health Service in the United Kingdom, did not employ an occupational therapist despite a clear role for the profession. I discussed the potential for occupational therapy in the service with the manager, and as I was also a senior lecturer at the time, I negotiated for them to host an occupational therapy student placement.

I was the liaison tutor providing weekly supervision. The placement went well, and the student worked on a one-to-one basis and researched, planned, delivered, and evaluated a group. At the end of the placement, she presented her work to a wide range of medical staff and managers, explaining the role and function of occupational therapy in the service. The feedback was amazing. Subsequently, funding was applied for, and nine months later a post was created. The now new graduate applied for the post and was successful in her appointment.

Alongside my senior lecturer role, I own a private service that provides professional supervision to over 80 occupational therapists nationally and internationally. I was asked to provide professional supervision for the new graduate, so I submitted a proposal to the management, and they agreed to fund monthly external supervision sessions.

That was back in 2009, fast-forward 12 years and that student occupational therapist is now working in the transgender clinic as a lead occupational therapist. She is recognised as an expert in her department and has two junior occupational therapists, whom she supervises.

In my view, the main strengths of external supervision were offering an outsider perspective to the strengths and areas for development within the organisation and providing consistency to maintain the vision and aims of the role throughout any periods of absence over the 12 years. Using Proctor's model (Proctor, 2001) to guide my supervision has also ensured that formative, normative, and restorative functions were addressed. This enabled us to successfully work together to create a new pathway embedding the occupational therapy process and achieving credible outcomes.

Continuing professional development for managers and leaders

The professional development needs of a manager or strategic leader, in our view, warrant separate consideration. As a strategic leader or manager, the level of your position and the functions of your role, which includes supervision of others, setting up supervision structures and educational opportunities, can leave you isolated in terms of sourcing appropriate non-line management supervision. Consideration is required for **how you will meet your own future growth and development goals, while being supported to stay connected to the profession** as well as develop as a professional leader and manager.

Many occupational therapy managers will be required to engage in operational supervision within their management role. This may include working on management skill development, career pathways, and project planning. Sustaining a connection to the profession may not be so readily available and may be best achieved through **connections to systems or peers outside of your employing organisation**. For example, some occupational therapy managers may prefer to organise peer supervision groups. In these groups you can arrange to meet regularly with fellow occupational therapists or health professional managers and strategic leaders who are at similar stages of their careers. In some countries the supervision needs of occupational therapy managers are being met through professional associations or systems set up for health professionals that are separate from those of their workplace, such as 'Mentorlink' by Occupational Therapy Australia (2021). These approaches rely on you **reaching a mutually crafted agreement for the supervision or partnership**. One potential conflict of interest here is that, when you approach others in similar position from different organisations to seek support, you may be approaching competitors that could be unable or unwilling to engage in a supervisory relationship. In such an instance, you may find alternative ways to seek support, and we have outlined some ideas in Chapter 8 where we discussed looking for supervision outside your organisation.

In the final section of this chapter, we will examine another key role of a manager in relation to supervision; how to evaluate the effectiveness of supervision processes and ways to build a case for quality improvement projects. These are topics in themselves which may warrant additional learning and support as you move into management roles, reinforcing the importance of Continuing development for the whole workforce.

MEASURING THE IMPACT OF SUPERVISION

The dynamic nature of supervision with varying perspectives on its purpose and benefits poses challenges to measuring its effectiveness and its contribution to individual and organisational outcomes. It also causes confusion about what is being measured, including those highlighted in **Box 9.13** (Martin et al., 2017).

BOX 9.13

Measuring effective supervision – what exactly are we measuring?

- Compliance with the preferred process of supervision in the organisation, such as completion rate of mandated professional performance and development plans?
- Supervisee contribution to supervision practices?
- Supervisee or supervisor satisfaction with supervision?
- Objective attainment of learning goals, or self-evaluation of goal attainment?
- All of the above?

Evaluation tasks of supervision practices have been reported to consist of two key components, namely summative practices and formative practices (Jones, 2006). **Summative evaluation** practices include formal assessment of supervision arrangements, the supervision alliance between the supervisor and supervisee, and change in the capability of the supervisee from their or the organisation's perspective. These formal evaluation practices typically use focus group interviews, semi-structured interviews, or self-reported questionnaires (Winstanley and White, 2003). Within some organisations people will be expected to engage in formal evaluation and complete necessary records for audit and quality assurance review. These may be reported and used as evidence of the service governance response to measure the impact of supervision at a strategic level across the organisation.

Formative evaluation practices tend to be more informal and may include feedback built into supervision including self-feedback by both parties, direct feedback to each party, feedback on the alliance, and any agreed goals and tasks forming the structure of supervision (Ducat and Kumar, 2015). It is likely that informal evaluation is part of the ongoing quality review of supervision, whereas the more formal summative approach to evaluation tends to occur less regularly and may potentially link directly to managerial practices or organisational assessment and appraisal functions.

In considering the evaluation of supervision we can also draw on evidence from exploring serious case incidents leading to major reviews that highlight the impact of what can go devastatingly wrong in a culture where supervision, learning, and support are inadequate.

As occupational therapists advance through their careers, self-evaluation becomes more important, especially when there are fewer peers and even fewer more senior members in career

TABLE 9.2 Examples of tools to measure supervision

Quality and effectiveness of supervision

- **The Manchester Clinical Supervision Scale (MCSS-26)** taps into supervisees' perceptions, supervisors' ability to discuss sensitive issues, to offer support, and to offer advice and guidance (Winstanley and White, 2014). The scale includes seven subscales which the supervisee rates and is based on Proctor's conceptual model of supervision.
- **Clinical Supervision Evaluation Questionnaire** (Horton et al., 2008) is a 14-item scale which rates overall perception of supervision in group supervision models which use a reflective process.

Supervisory relationship

- **Supervisory Relationship Questionnaire** (Paloma et al., 2010) is a 67-item scale completed by the supervisee to evaluate their perspective of the supervisory relationship.

Supervisory style

- **The Supervisory Styles Inventory** (Friedlander and Ward, 1984) is a 33-item scale which can be used by both supervisor and supervisee. The outcomes indicate the perceived supervisory style in the categories 'attractive', 'interpersonally sensitive', and 'task-oriented'.

Supervisor self-rating

- **The Clinical Supervision Self-Assessment Tool** is based on the National Clinical Supervision Competency Resource developed by Health Workforce Australia (2013). This tool is for the supervisor to self-rate their clinical supervisor skills, knowledge, and confidence.

Direct observation of supervision

- **Supervision: Adherence and Guidance Evaluation (SAGE)** is a 23-item, direct observation instrument, developed to meet the growing need for competence monitoring and evaluation in cognitive behavioural therapy supervision. The Short-SAGE, a revised version, is a 14-item version of SAGE (Reiser et al., 2018).

structures. For example, occupational therapists who are chief executives of organisations or in senior strategic roles are functioning as experts. As a profession, it is important for us to consider how we support these members of our occupational therapy community to continue to grow.

There is a range of tools available to measure aspects of supervision. It is first helpful to consider what you want to use the results for, so you can determine which aspect of supervision evaluation would best meet your needs. As a starting point, **Table 9.2** offers some examples.

We began this chapter by outlining the benefits of supervision to organisations and we have ended it with a brief exploration of some of the measures that can be used to capture the impact of it. Underlying all of the elements that we have discussed is the need for managerial and strategic leadership support to embed supervision into the day-to-day activities of the workplace.

CRITICAL COMMENTARY

The value placed on supervision

This chapter has explored some of the factors to be considered at managerial and strategic leadership levels to support the development of effective supervisory practice. It is not exhaustive, and further considerations will be needed as new roles and new ways of working emerge within the workforce. For example, in the United Kingdom, it has been proposed that multi-professional advanced practitioners have several supervisors – one for educational development, one for professional practice development, and one for profession-specific sources of support (Health Education England, 2020).

There are several topics for us to consider, some more than others depending on what already exists within your own work context. For example, should the occupational therapy profession recommend several different supervisors and move to separate line management responsibility from professional development support? Do we need to look at a different model of supervision to ensure all aspects are balanced equitably and we can respond to the changing nature of our workplaces? What capabilities exist in the team to write business plans to support change? Is there sufficient representation at organisational and strategic levels to support the development of supervision practices? Some organisations have established practice development lead roles, where the person in post works across the health professions to embed processes such as supervision into the wider systems.

Fundamental to addressing these questions, and highlighted in Helen's work, is the need for a deeper understanding of the value placed on supervision at the organisational, managerial, and individual levels so we can strive to improve and develop inclusive practices.

SUMMARY

In this chapter, we have brought the 3Cs back together and applied them to managerial and strategic levels within organisations. The duality of roles and balancing the needs of the organisation with the needs of the supervisee were explored, alongside illustrative examples and suggestions on how tensions could be navigated.

We returned to the importance of the supervisory relationship and argued that inclusive supervision needs to be driven from a strategic level, ensuring there are policies, processes, and structures in place to provide the right conditions. Ongoing learning and development for supervisors was recognised alongside the need for strategic leaders to find their own development opportunities too.

Supervision is critical for public and professional safety, so this chapter addressed ways to evaluate it in practice and to engage in a process of continued quality improvement. The recommended starting point was to explore the value placed on supervision within the organisation you work in, so initiatives to improve the delivery are pitched at the right level. Once this has been done, then plans can be made on how to make changes in practice. Our final chapter will offer a framework to support change into practice as part of developing plans for action.

REFERENCES

Brown, R., Desai, S., and Elliott, C., (2019). *Identity-conscious supervision in student affairs: building relationships and transforming systems.* Abingdon: Routledge.

Busari, J.O. and Koot, B.G. (2007) 'Quality of clinical supervision as perceived by attending doctors in university and district teaching hospitals', *Medical Education*, 41, pp. 957–964. doi:10.1111/j.1365-2923.2007.02837.x

Dancza, K., Choi, Y.M., Amalia, K., Wong, P.S., Hu, J.H., and Yap, L.W. (2021) 'An appreciative inquiry approach to understanding what attracts and retains early-career therapists to work in community organizations', *The Internet Journal of Allied Health Sciences and Practice*, 20(1), pp. 1–13. 10.46743/1540-580X/2022.2002.

Dawson, P.M. (2003). *Understanding organisational change: the contemporary experience of people at work.* London: SAGE.

Deci, E.L. and Ryan, R.M. (2010). 'Self-determination', in Weiner, I.B. and Craighead, W.E. (eds) (2010). *The Corsini encyclopedia of psychology.* Hoboken, NJ: John Wiley.

Ducat, W.H. and Kumar, S. (2015) 'A systematic review of professional supervision experiences and effects for allied health practitioners working in non-metropolitan health care settings', *Journal of Multidisciplinary Healthcare*, 8, pp. 397–407. doi:10.2147/JMDH.S84557.

Evaluation Works (n.d.) National Health Service evaluation cycle. Available at: https://nhsevaluationtoolkit. net/evaluation-cycle/ (Accessed: 19 March 2021).

Friedlander, M.L. and Ward, L.G. (1984) 'Development and validation of the Supervisory Styles Inventory', *Journal of Counseling Psychology*, 31(4), pp. 541–557. doi:10.1037/0022-0167.31.4.541.

Health and Care Professions Council (2020) *The characteristics of effective supervision.* London: Health and Care Professions Council. Available at: www.hcpc-uk.org/resources/reports/2019/effective-clinical-and-peer-supervision-report/ (Accessed: 8 May 2021).

Health Education England (2020) *Workplace supervision for advanced clinical practice: an integrated multi-professional approach for practitioner development.* Available at: www.hee.nhs.uk/our-work/advanced-practice/reports-publications/workplace-supervision-advanced-clinical-practice (Accessed: 31 May 2021).

Health Workforce Australia (2013) *National clinical supervision competency resource – validation edition.* Available at: http://www.clinedaus.org.au/files/resources/hwa_national_clinical_supervision_competency_resource_ve_201305_2.pdf (Accessed: 26 September 2021).

Horton, S., Drachler, M.D.L., Fuller, A., and Leite, J.C.D.C. (2008) 'Development and preliminary validation of a measure for assessing staff perspectives on the quality of clinical group supervision', *International Journal of Language and Communication Disorders*, 43(2), pp. 126–134. doi:10.1080/13682820701380031.

Jones, A. (2006) 'Clinical supervision: what do we know and what do we need to know? A review and commentary', *Journal of Nursing Management*, 14(8), pp. 577–585. doi:10.1111/j.1365-2934.2006.00716.x.

Kramer-Roy, D., Hashim, D., Tahir, N., Khan, A., Khalid, A., Faiz, N., Minai, R., Jawaid, S., Khan, S., Rashid, R., and Frater, T. (2020) 'The developing role of occupational therapists in school-based practice: experiences from collaborative action research in Pakistan', *British Journal of Occupational Therapy*, 83(6), pp. 375–386. doi:10.1177/0308022619891841.

Martin, P., Kumar, S., and Lizarondo, L. (2017) 'Effective use of technology in clinical supervision', *Internet Interventions*, 8, pp. 35–39. doi:10.1016/j.invent.2017.03.001.

Nancarrow, S.A., Wade, R., Moran, M., Coyle, J., Young, J., and Boxall, D. (2014) 'Connecting practice: a practitioner centred model of supervision', *Clinical Governance: An International Journal*, 19(3), pp. 235–253. doi:10.1108/CGIJ-03-2014-0010.

Occupational Therapy Australia (2019) *Professional supervision framework.* Melbourne: Occupational Therapy Australia.

Occupational Therapy Australia (2021) *Mentorlink programme.* Available at: https://otaus.com.au/membership/ota-member-programs/mentorlink (Accessed: 26 September 2021).

Pack, M. (2015) '"Unsticking the stuckness": a qualitative study of the clinical supervisory needs of early-career health social workers', *British Journal of Social Work*, 45(6), pp. 1821–1836. doi:10.1093/bjsw/bcu069.

Paloma, M., Beinart, H., and Cooper, M. (2010) 'Development and validation of the Supervisory Relationship Questionnaire (SRQ) in UK clinical trainees', *British Journal of Clinical Psychology*, 49, pp. 131–149.

Proctor, B. (2001) 'Training for the supervision alliance attitude, skills and intention', in Cutcliffe, J.R., Butterworth, T., and Proctor, B. (eds) *Fundamental themes in clinical supervision.* London: Routledge, pp. 25–46.

Reiser, R.P., Cliffe, T., and Milne, D.L. (2018) 'An improved competence rating scale for CBT Supervision: Short-SAGE', *The Cognitive Behaviour Therapist*, 11, pp. 1–16. doi:10.1017/S1754470X18000065.

Rice, D.B., Taylor, R., and Forrester, J.K. (2020) 'The unwelcoming experience of abusive supervision and the impact of leader characteristics: turning employees into poor organizational citizens and future quitters', *European Journal of Work and Organizational Psychology*, 29(4), pp. 601–618. doi:10.1080/13594 32X.2020.1737521.

Singh, A. and Chun, K.Y.S. (2010) '"From the margins to the center": moving towards a resilience-based model of supervision for queer people of color supervisors', *Training and Education in Professional Psychology*, 4(1), pp. 36–46. doi:10.1037/a0017373.

Think Pacific. 2020. The 5D internship journey. Available at: https://thinkpacific.com/remote-internships-scholarship-program (Accessed: 27 March 2022).

Winstanley, J. and White, E. (2003) 'Clinical supervision: models, measures and best practice', *Nurse Researcher*, 10(4), pp. 7–38.

Winstanley, J., and White, E. (2014). The Manchester Clinical Supervision Scale©: MCSS-26©. In Watkins, C.E., Jr. & Milne, D.L. (eds) *The Wiley Blackwell international handbook of clinical supervision*. Chichester: Wiley Blackwell, pp. 386–401. doi:10.1002/9781118846360.ch17.

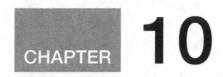

10

Creating change and future directions in supervision

Stephanie Tempest, Karina Dancza, and Anita Volkert

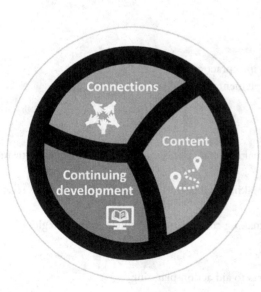

Connections
The active process of nurturing and maintaining supervisory relationships

Content
The topics and structures that guide supervision

Continuing development
The enhancement of knowledge and skills to be a capable occupational therapist and effective supervisor/supervisee

DOI: 10.4324/9781003092544-10

CHAPTER INTENTIONS

In this chapter we invite you to:

* Examine the unanswered questions about supervision to inform future research
* Appraise selected approaches to implement change in practice
* Consider our intentions for ongoing work to support effective supervision
* Formulate an action plan to enhance your effectiveness as a supervisor and/or supervisee.

CHAPTER HIGHLIGHTS

* Planning a way forward for supervision
* Supervision and the need for more research
* How to introduce change drawing from implementation science
* And finally (nearly!): What would you like to do next?
* Critical commentary: Our aspirations for supervision

CHAPTER RESOURCES

Figures

* Figure 10.1 The leaky pipeline of ideas into practice
* Figure 10.2 Six Steps from Ideas to Implementation

Tables

* Table 10.1 Facilitators and barriers to making change and implementation strategies relating to capability
* Table 10.2 Facilitators and barriers to making change and implementation strategies relating to opportunity
* Table 10.3 Facilitators and barriers to making change and implementation strategies relating to motivation
* Table 10.4 Implementation outcomes
* Table 10.5 Overview of chapter contents to aid action planning

Boxes

* Box 10.1 Unanswered research questions for supervision
* Box 10.2 Illustrative example: Formulating ideas for changes to supervisory practices
* Box 10.3 Seven Ps to categorise changes
* Box 10.4 Discussion questions for refining the 'what' and 'who' of making a change
* Box 10.5 Discussion questions for refining the barriers and facilitators for making a change

- Box 10.6 Example ways to gather outcome data
- Box 10.7 Ideas for sustaining change

Appendices

- Appendix 10.1 Six Steps from Ideas to Implementation guidance template
- Appendix 10.2 Actions to enhance supervision guidance template

PLANNING A WAY FORWARD FOR SUPERVISION

In this, our final chapter, we would like to look to the future with you. We will focus on three areas, sharing our thoughts about research priorities for supervision, creating change to supervisory practices, and inviting you to reflect on your own priorities and engagement in needed actions.

First, we will propose a list of research questions which we feel are the main priorities going forward. We welcome your thoughts and hope you will add to them too. Some of the research questions have been identified through systematic processes (and their sources have been acknowledged), and some of the questions have emerged from our experiences, including through engaging in many conversations and the process of writing this book.

Second, because we are pragmatic realists, we want to briefly explore methods to support change to supervisory processes within practice. We all have different reactions to change, and indeed those reactions change themselves depending on what is going on for us at that moment in time. Therefore, we need to introduce any changes to supervision practice in an intentional and planned way.

Once explored, we bring this book to a close by inviting you to come with us to formulate action plans. We are keen to identify things that we can do to enhance supervision within the next week, month, year, and longer, no matter how big or small the changes may be. So, let's get started by talking about research.

SUPERVISION AND THE NEED FOR MORE RESEARCH

We know that stating the need for more research in an area is an all too familiar sentiment, as we are yet to find an area of our practice where we can say 'we have all the research we need!'. However, we would like to frame this as an exciting opportunity and a challenge that we can embrace. We also want to offer reassurance that we are not at the starting line either, as there is work already underway within and beyond our profession.

We know that while there are positive associations between supervision and meaningful outcomes (see Chapter 9), there is limited research evidence to support the effectiveness of supervision within occupational therapy (Occupational Therapy Australia, 2019). This may be because supervision has not yet attracted much interest and research funding, combined with the complexity of designing robust supervision research studies. However, in a systematic review, Snowdon et al. (2017)

found that 'processes' of care associated with enhanced health outcomes for people who access services, were significantly improved because health professionals engaged in supervision. And in a mixed methods systematic review, Martin et al., (2021) concluded that supervision could mitigate the risk of burnout, facilitate staff retention, and improve the work environment. They also found evidence to show that inadequate supervision was harmful and can lead to stress and burnout. So, we owe it to ourselves and the people who access our services to develop the evidence base for supervision.

Research into supervision has expanded in the last decade in counselling, psychotherapy, psychology, nursing, and social work, and we have drawn on this throughout the book. However, while steadily growing, the evolving research continues to have limitations. One-off research designs continue to dominate, and further, longitudinal work is needed to explore a range of questions, for example, the impact of effective supervision on professional development. The focus also tends to be on the supervisee experience and while this is not wrong, there is further work to understand supervision from the supervisors' and wider organisational perspectives. Enhancing effective supervision practices requires us to understand it from multiple viewpoints so we can accurately identify enablers and barriers and enact change.

Five key areas of emerging and future research in supervision practice have been identified by Hawkins and McMahon (2020). Additionally, within **Box 10.1** we have added our own thoughts on specific, unanswered questions within occupational therapy supervision. The list is by no means exhaustive, and you are invited to consider additional questions, too.

BOX 10.1

Unanswered research questions for supervision

Future research key areas (Hawkins and McMahon, 2020)

1. How do people who access services benefit from professionals attending supervision?
2. How does supervision contribute to professional capability and career development?
3. What is the impact of supervision on staff retention, wellbeing, and resilience, including stress and burnout?
4. What are the problematic issues in supervision?
5. What are good supervision practices?

Our own additional questions

- Can the 3Cs for Effective Supervision support supervisory processes at individual, organisational, and strategic levels?
- Can appreciative, strengths-based supervisory approaches enhance experiences of supervision for supervisors and supervisees?

- How can we make supervision more inclusive?
- To what extent does supervision support supervisees working with high levels of complexity?
- Is remote/telesupervision as effective as face-to-face methods?
- What further education is needed for supervisors, and how do we know if it is effective?
- How do we improve supervisory processes in organisations, including at a strategic level?
- What is the outcome of embedding supervisory strategies to support the workforce?
- To what extent does supervision contribute to public and professional safety?
- How can we bring about change to enhance supervisory practices?

We would love to hear your thoughts on future research questions for supervision (e.g. by using **#3CSupervision** on social media to keep this conversation going). We have really appreciated all the stories of supervisory practices shared with us from the contributors in this book, and we would also be very interested in your stories about what you have already done or your plans for supervision. Future editions of this book may look very different if we are able to collect and share stories of supervision research projects undertaken within the profession. Stories that make it to publication are fantastic, but to build a critical mass, we can also bring smaller projects and ideas together.

With a defined list of the starting points for future research, we would like to turn our attention to how we can make changes to current supervisory practices, using what we already know from our existing research, knowledge, skills, and experiences, such as those we have shared throughout this book. Dissemination and implementation of findings is the final part of the research process and it is as essential as all other steps in the research cycle. However, because implementing change is so complex, it has also become a scientific discipline in its own right. The next section will provide a brief overview of how to introduce change into practice, drawing on the evidence base to do so.

HOW TO INTRODUCE CHANGE DRAWING FROM IMPLEMENTATION SCIENCE

Introducing new ideas into practice is not straightforward, and making changes to supervision is no exception. Although not directly related to supervision, studies have shown that 40–45% of new initiatives fail to maintain the proposed change, and more than half do not continue the change at high levels of fidelity (Scheireret et al., 2005; Stirmanet et al., 2012). The challenge is that unless the change is seen as usual practice, interest is likely to fade when we are faced with new or competing priorities (Dixon-Woods et al., 2012; Ling et al., 2010).

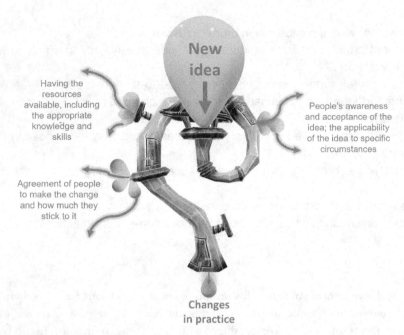

Having the
resources
available, including
the appropriate
knowledge and
skills

New
idea

People's awareness
and acceptance of the
idea; the applicability
of the idea to specific
circumstances

Agreement of people
to make the change
and how much they
stick to it

Changes
in practice

FIGURE 10.1 The leaky pipeline of ideas into practice (adapted from Glasziou and Haynes, 2005)

We know from work on evidence-based practice that there is a "leaky pipeline" (Glasziou and Haynes, 2005, p. 37) between new ideas and evidence making its way into what we are doing **(Figure 10.1)**. We may also refer to this as a theory-to-practice gap. Leakage can occur if people are **not aware** of the new idea or **do not accept** the idea as important or relevant to them. Further leaks happen when people **do not have the resources, knowledge, skills, or confidence** to carry out the idea. Sometimes the idea has **not been well developed or described** so it is difficult to use. Finally, the leaks can occur if people **do not agree** with the change, or it is **tried and abandoned** at the first setback or when the initial excitement or support fades (Glasziou and Haynes, 2005).

Attempting to make a change to practice without a theoretically driven strategy is a costly game of trial and error (Nilsen, 2015). To address this, whole areas of research have been created such as implementation science, knowledge translation, and quality improvement approaches (Wensing and Grol, 2019). **Figure 10.2** provides an overview of six key steps in designing a strategy for implementing a new idea and **Appendix 10.1** offers a guidance template (see also Handley et al., 2016). If you are interested to explore this body of knowledge further, here are a few implementation design process models that could be useful:

- Knowledge-to-Action (Graham et al., 2006)
- Exploration Preparation Implementation Sustainment (EPIS) Implementation Framework (Aarons et al., 2011; Moullin et al., 2019)
- Intervention Mapping (Bartholomew Eldredge et al., 2016)
- The Hexagon Tool: Exploring Context (Metz and Louison, 2018)

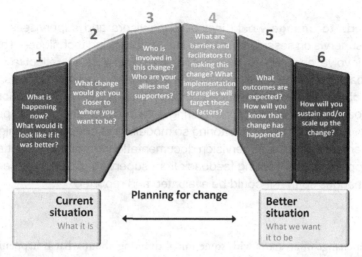

FIGURE 10.2 Six Steps from Ideas to Implementation (adapted from Moore and Khan, 2020)

Step 1: What is happening now? What would it look like if it was better?

When thinking about change, it is helpful to consider what is currently happening and what it would look like if it was better or improved in some way. When introducing a change in supervision, think about two important concepts: **(1) what needs to change, and (2) how to make the change**. We invite you to read the following illustrative example where a manager begins thinking about making a change to supervisory practices **(Box 10.2)**.

BOX 10.2

Illustrative example: Formulating ideas for changes to supervisory practices

Reflecting on Chapter 7 and how we can apply our occupational therapy perspectives to supervision, I wondered how I could plan for a coaching approach to be introduced at a service level to enhance supervision. Our team collaboratively reviewed the literature about using an appreciative, strengths-based approach and coaching techniques, and together we decided there was enough evidence to apply some strategies to enhance our supervision practices. Here are our initial thoughts about what needed to change and how we could implement change:

> **What needs to change** would include supervisors and supervisees adapting their supervision session formats to include coaching techniques. This would also involve changes to the supervision paperwork to reflect a coaching approach, requiring adjustment to the administration arrangements.
>
> **How the change will be introduced** could be through running education events on coaching for supervisors; pairing experienced and less experienced supervisors together for mentoring so modelling of coaching techniques can happen; updating the supervision documentation formats to reflect a coaching approach; and seeking feedback from supervisor and supervisees about the changes so that it could be evaluated and reported.

Making a change often starts with some initial thinking about what is happening now and what it would look like if it was improved. As highlighted in the illustrative example, this is a good start, but it will need refinement to bring effective and sustainable changes into practice. So, once an initial idea is formed, it is time to identify specifics and think about what has informed your decisions so far.

Step 2: What change would get you closer to where you want to be?

From your initial idea, clarify exactly what people will do differently by making an explicit list of required changes. This will build on your initial thinking about what needs to change. Brown et al. (2017) suggested the 7 Ps to categories changes **(Box 10.3)** and you may find you need a combination of things to change to make a sustainable difference to practice.

BOX 10.3

7 Ps to categorise changes (adapted from Brown et al., 2017)

1. **Programs:** A set of coordinated activities to accomplish a specific goal (e.g. a prepackaged evidence-based programme, such as the use of Occupational Performance Coaching for supervisors to use in supervision (Graham et al., 2020).
2. **Practices:** The application of an idea or belief (e.g. monitoring the use of guideline recommendations for group supervision, or the use of coaching questions).
3. **Policies:** Legislative/regulatory decisions made to ensure that specific actions can be taken within a legal/regulatory framework (e.g. policies about minimum standards for supervision).

4. **Procedures:** A set of instructions or sequential activities that help guide a specific action (e.g. use of supervision outcome measures).
5. **Principles:** Beliefs/philosophies that guide action (e.g. using an appreciative, strengths-based approach in supervision).
6. **Pills:** Refers broadly to any drugs that might be used to improve outcomes (e.g. medication – maybe not so relevant to supervision!).
7. **Products:** Tools or resources that guide people in accomplishing activities/goals (e.g. an online learning platform, electronic supervision records, or mobile phone applications to monitor supervision and professional development).

In the earlier illustrative example, we could define the introduction of a coaching approach in supervision as requiring (1) a **change in practices** (using coaching questions to guide supervision), (2) a **change in principles** (framing supervision interactions using an appreciative, strengths-based approach), and (3) a **change in procedures** (using a new supervision documentation format reflecting a coaching approach).

Step 3: Who is involved in this change? Who are your allies and supporters?

Once you are aware of what exactly needs to change, your attention can turn to who will be involved in creating and sustaining these changes. This will differ depending on your setting, but may include:

- Supervisors: May need to do something differently (e.g. a new supervisory procedure, outcome measurement, using group supervision, approaching supervision from an appreciative, strengths-based perspective, etc.)
- Supervisees: May need to accept something different (e.g. group supervision, supervision from someone who is not an occupational therapist, a more active role in supervision if a coaching approach is adopted, etc.)
- Administrators/managers: May need to create new systems or use different processes to support the change (e.g. shared time for group supervision, new documentation formats, systems for allocating/selecting supervisors and supervisees, processes for resolving conflict, etc.)
- Others: There may be other stakeholders such as linked services or the people who access services who need to do something differently or will be affected by the change.

It is also vital to consider who are your allies and supporters for this change. Change can be exciting, but also uncomfortable and challenging, so take care of yourself by having people around you that you can turn to when needed. Pausing to get the initial steps as comprehensive as possible will be beneficial before moving on. **Box 10.4** suggests some questions you may wish to think about and review with relevant stakeholders.

> **BOX 10.4**
>
> **Discussion questions for refining the 'what' and 'who' of making a change**
>
> - Who are the key stakeholders who will make the decision about the proposed change? Is it possible to arrange a discussion with the relevant people?
> - What is the change that is proposed? How does it relate to the 7 Ps?
> - What is the rationale and evidence for the effectiveness of the proposed change?
> - Is the proposed change clearly defined and realistic given the current situation (small changes may be more easily introduced and sustained)?
> - Who will need to make a change?
> - Who is best placed to understand what the day-to-day reality is like for the people who will make the change?
> - What supports can I draw on to drive this change?
> - Who are my allies or people I can turn to for guidance and support?

Step 4: What are the barriers and facilitators to making this change? What implementation strategies will target these factors?

When seeking to make a change, we often rely on tried and tested measures for driving change, for example hosting a workshop or an awareness campaign. While these implementation strategies may be effective if people require greater knowledge or awareness to make the change happen, if the barriers for change are something else, then these strategies can miss the mark. Investing time to find out what the facilitators and barriers are for making a change, then targeting your implementation strategies to address these factors increases the likelihood of success. **Information could be sourced from conducting a literature review, interviewing, or surveying relevant stakeholders or through informal discussions**.

Once you know more about the barriers and facilitators to change, it can be useful to map these onto a framework or theory of behaviour change to understand what is happening and so you can select an appropriate implementation strategy. For example, the COM-B Model and Theoretical Domains Framework (Atkins et al., 2017) suggests that **making a change in behaviour (B) requires three things: the person needs to be capable of change (C), have the opportunity to change (O), and be motivated to change (M)**, and these factors can be applied to organisations too.

Supporting people to change their behaviour is not new to us as occupational therapists. When we work with people accessing our services, we often consider and use similar theories to support change to enable occupational performance and participation, although we may call it 'professional reasoning'. So, our intention is to invite you to consider using knowledge and skills that you already have in identifying barriers and facilitators and linking appropriate implementation strategies to create change in supervision practices. To illustrate, we will discuss how each of the elements in COM-B and Theoretical Domains Framework (Atkins et al., 2017) could be useful when considering how to address barriers and leverage facilitators of change. To begin, **Table 10.1** unpacks when the facilitators or barriers are related to **capability** and suggests relevant implementation strategies. **Table 10.2** then outlines potential facilitators, barriers, and implementation strategies related to **opportunity** in supervision. Finally, **Table 10.3** outlines facilitators, barriers, and implementation strategies for change related to **motivation** in supervision.

TABLE 10.1 Facilitators and barriers to making change and implementation strategies relating to capability

Capability	
Theoretical Domains Framework subsections	Examples
Knowledge An awareness that something exists	• People's level of familiarity with roles and responsibilities of supervision; supervision frameworks; different supervisory approaches (such as peer, group, or interprofessional supervision). • Implementation strategies for enhancing knowledge are educational and could include learning materials, workshops, communities of practice, etc.
Skills An ability to do something capably, usually acquired through practice	• People's level of skill in questioning, active listening, reflection, coaching, or creative activities to meet supervisory demands. • Implementation strategies for enhancing skills focus on learning and development opportunities where practice and feedback are available.
Memory, attention, decision processes The ability to recall information, focus selectively on tasks, and choose between two or more alternatives	• People's recall of supervisory requirements, details, timing, recording of procedures, or responsibilities. • Implementation strategies to address challenges relating to memory, attention, and decision processes may be external reminders such as calendar applications, reinforcement in team meetings, periodic reminders to complete supervision paperwork, or protocols and reflective strategies to support decision making.

(Continued)

TABLE 10.1 (Continued)

Capability	
Theoretical Domains Framework subsections	**Examples**
Behavioural regulation Anything aimed at managing or changing actions	• People's established ways of doing supervision and how these ways are embedded in the service. Introducing a new supervisory approach may mean letting go of something established to make space for the new activity and embedding new habits. • Implementation strategies may be educational but could also include modelling of the approach by identified champions or encouragement/reinforcement/incentivisation by peers, colleagues, and managers.

(adapted from Atkins et al., 2017; Moore and Khan, 2020)

TABLE 10.2 Facilitators and barriers to making change and implementation strategies relating to opportunity

Opportunity	
Theoretical Domains Framework subsections	**Examples**
Environmental and contextual resources Anything in the situation or context that helps or hinders the performance of a person	• Resources could include time for supervision, a private space for supervision, funds to attend relevant educational courses, availability of supervisors or mentors in the setting, and many other things. • Implementation strategies to address environmental and contextual constraints may include making changes to schedules, creating private spaces in the setting, or seeking funding and leveraging existing knowledge and skills for educational opportunities.
Social influences The relationships or influences that can cause people to change their thoughts, feelings, or behaviours	• People's experiences of relationships, prior experiences of supervision, how supervision is viewed and valued by colleagues, the culture of the workplace, what others in the setting are saying about supervision can influence how supervision and change are accepted. • Implementation strategies when social influences are negatively impacting on how supervision functions would aim to change the social environment. For example, seeking a mandate for supervision from management, identifying supervision champions who will drive the change or leveraging local, national, or international policies and best practice guidelines for supervision. Supervision policies and a culture that recognises the benefits and potential harms of supervision may also be helpful.

(adapted from Atkins et al., 2017; Moore and Khan, 2020)

TABLE 10.3 Facilitators and barriers to making change and implementation strategies relating to motivation

Motivation	
Theoretical Domains Framework subsections	**Examples**
Beliefs about capabilities How you feel about your ability to do something constructive	• People's views of their expertise to engage with supervision. • Implementation strategies to encourage people to have more agency over what they do could include education, mentoring/peer support, modelling, encouragement/reinforcement/incentivisation by peers, colleagues, and managers.
Beliefs about consequences Anticipation of what will happen if something is done or not done	• People's anticipation (e.g. fear, excitement, exhaustion) of what will happen if something changes in the way supervision is done. Beliefs about consequences are likely influenced by people's prior experiences of supervision and how positive or negative they were. • Implementation strategies when people believe something negative could result from the change may include education, mentoring/peer support, modelling, encouragement/reassurance/reinforcement/incentivisation by peers, colleagues, and managers.
Social/professional role and identity How you behave and think of yourself as belonging to a social or professional group	• How people view being a supervisor or supervisee as part of their work role or professional identity (e.g. 'It's not my job', or 'It is part of who I am'). • Implementation strategies when people do not see supervision as part of their role could include education, modelling, workplace policy or job description changes, encouragement/reinforcement/incentivisation by peers, colleagues, and managers.
Optimism/pessimism The confidence that things will be possible or not	• People's perception of the impact proposed changes will have on professional practice, or the work being done. • Implementation strategies when people are not confident that changes to supervision will make a difference could include education, refinement/clarity of the proposed change, modelling, or supervision champions to persuade people of the value of the change.
Intentions A conscious aim or plan to do something	• People's perception or understanding of the value of the proposed changes to the supervisory arrangements and the likelihood that they will take the necessary steps to do things differently. • Implementation strategies when people do not commit to making a change could include making the change a visible part of the workload (e.g. through key performance indicators or audit), or considering the wider work of people and trying to address how to balance requirements and create space for change.

(Continued)

TABLE 10.3 (Continued)

	Motivation	
Theoretical Domains Framework subsections	**Examples**	
Goals An outcome that a person wants to achieve	• People's perception that changes to supervision align with their personal or professional goals and their willingness to work towards them. • Implementation strategies could include collaboration and co-creation of the supervisory changes with supervisors and supervisees, offering choice and control in changes and implementation strategies, and incentivisation through linking goals with workload measures and appraisal performance.	
Emotion A complex reaction as a person attempts to deal with a personally significant matter or event	• People's emotional reactions to supervision potentially related to prior experiences, both positive and negative. People's perceived safety of the supervisory process to be open and express vulnerability in supervision to facilitate learning. People's perception of their effectiveness of doing existing practices and if change is taken personally. • Implementation strategies when emotional reactions are a barrier for change could include making policy changes so that the culture of supervision recognises power differences and supports accountability for actions. Modelling supervisory practices and mentoring/peer support could also be helpful.	
Reinforcement Enhancing the likelihood of something happening by introducing a stimulus	• People's willingness to change if offered appropriate incentives such as career progression, recognition, educational opportunities, more money, or disincentives such as restrictions in their career progression, limits to their job scope, or being performance managed. • Implementation strategies when people view external reinforcement as a reason for change could include incentives such as consideration of supervision undertaken in appraisals or rewards for excellence in supervisory practices. Reinforcement could also be negative, and people not adhering to the change may experience consequences in performance reviews or restrictions placed on practices. Adherence could be monitored via audit and feedback.	

(adapted from Atkins et al., 2017; Moore and Khan, 2020)

We have highlighted how we can plan our implementation strategies to target specific barriers and leverage facilitators. For a refined compilation of implementation strategies from the Expert Recommendations for Implementing Change (ERIC) project, please see Powell et al. (2015). Having a targeted plan may mean greater success in introducing change and hopefully less wasted effort. **Box 10.5** suggests some questions for refining implementation ideas and could be useful to stimulate discussion with relevant stakeholders.

BOX 10.5

Discussion questions for refining the barriers and facilitators for making a change

- What do we already know about the barriers and facilitators to introducing a change in this context? How do we know this?
- What do we know from the literature about potential barriers and facilitators to making this type of change?
- Who else do we need to ask to understand other potential issues in implementing this change?
- How do we plan on asking people about what they perceive are the barriers and facilitators to making this change (e.g. team meeting, survey, focus group, semi-structured interviews, etc.)?

Step 5: What outcomes are expected? How will you know change has happened?

Measuring outcomes is standard practice in many areas of occupational therapy. When planning a change, it is important to consider how you will measure if change has been introduced and maintained (Proctor et al., 2015). Some important aspects when considering sustainability of a change are resources that were used; demonstrating effectiveness of the change; monitoring the change over time; involvement and participation from relevant stakeholders; and how the change has integrated within existing programmes and policies. The **RE-AIM framework** (Reach, Effectiveness, Adoption, Implementation, and Maintenance) is another commonly used tool for outcome evaluation planning (Glasgow et al., 1999, 2019). **Table 10.4** presents a range of outcomes that you may wish to consider (Proctor et al., 2011), and **Box 10.6** suggests ways to gather this information.

TABLE 10.4 Implementation outcomes

Outcome	Description	When it is most useful
Acceptability	Perception that the change (e.g. content, complexity, delivery, credibility) is satisfactory	• Early adopters • Ongoing monitoring (penetration) • Year-on-year sustainability
Adoption	Intention to try, decision to do, or action to take up the change and use it in practice	• Early-to-mid project cycle
Appropriateness	Perceived fit, relevance, suitability, usefulness, or compatibility of the change within the context or to address a specific issue	• Prior to adoption/introduction of the change

(Continued)

TABLE 10.4 (Continued)

Outcome	Description	When it is most useful
Feasibility	The extent to which the change can be successfully used or delivered in a context	• Early project cycle during the initial adoption of the change
Fidelity	The extent to which the change is delivered as originally intended and adheres to the recommended plans or protocols	• Early-to-mid project cycle
Implementation cost	How much the change will cost to be implemented	• Early for adoption and feasibility Mid for penetration Late for sustainability
Penetration	How much the change has spread within the context or how much the change has reached its target population	• Mid-to-late project cycle
Sustainability	The extent to which the change has been maintained and become habitual in the context	• Late project cycle

(adapted from Proctor et al., 2011)

BOX 10.6

Example ways to gather outcome data

- Surveys
- Semi-structured interviews
- Focus groups
- Staff meeting minutes
- Informal feedback (will need to be captured in some way)
- Audit of notes or other administrative processes
- Amount of uptake/refusal to change
- Administrative data (e.g. expenses, time given to the change, number of people involved, etc.)
- Outputs such as number/frequency of people trained, accessing a resource, inputting to a new system, etc.
- Observations
- Self-reports
- Checklists

Step 6: How will you sustain and/or scale up the change?

Steps 1–5 described how to plan for creating a change in supervisory practices. Step 6 moves from this design phase to consider how to carry out the **implementation of the change**, how the changes may **spread** (an organic process as people take up new ideas on their own) and **scale-up** of change (a deliberate process of introducing the change beyond the initial context) (Moore and Khan, 2020). There are additional process models that take you through this phase, including **Getting to Outcomes (GTO)** (Chinman et al., 2008) and **Quality Implementation Framework (QIF)** (Meyers et al., 2012).

When considering how the change will be implemented, there are many contextual factors that could offer insights into how and why people take up a new idea or not. In addition, people may be at different stages of readiness for change. While many implementation efforts fail because people are not ready for change, being ready does not guarantee success either. The **Consolidated Framework for Implementation Research (CFIR)** (Damschroder et al., 2009) offers a way to think through characteristics of the inner and outer setting to understand how they impact on implementation and outcomes, and may be helpful as you embark on creating change. Some additional ideas for implementing change are offered in **Box 10.7**.

BOX 10.7

Ideas for sustaining change

- As occupational therapists, we are familiar with the importance of **routines in sustaining a change**. Embedding changes in supervisory practices in organisational routines, paperwork, and workplace cultures could encourage sustainability of new practices.
- Acknowledging that people like to put their own perspectives on new ideas, **anticipating that adaptations to the new practices will happen and intentionally guiding this process**, helps people accept change while maintaining the effective features of the change.
- Thinking back to the leaky pipeline, where new ideas can take up to 17 years to embed in practice, we have some evidence that with a dedicated **implementation team**, we can create change in just three years (Balas and Boren, 2000). An implementation team consists of people who help to drive the change, guides people to use the new strategies, and works through implementation challenges as they arise.

We are now at the stage where we have considered research questions which may help our understanding and implementation of supervisory practices in the future, and then explored an intentional way to implement change into practice. The next logical step is to identify the things you would like to attempt to change in your own practice, remembering that sometimes change can happen one conversation at a time.

AND FINALLY (NEARLY!): WHAT WOULD YOU LIKE TO DO NEXT?

As we draw this chapter and indeed this book to a close, we invite you to take some time to think about what actions you want to take to enhance the effectiveness of yourself as a supervisee, as a supervisor, and/or the development of practices at operational or strategic levels. Think about what is within your sphere of influence. For example, would you consider a conversation about using creative methods within your supervision? And if so, who would you have this conversation with and what would you like to see happen within your own service?

To help you do this, we invite you to think about actions you would like to set yourself linked to the content of each chapter (see **Table 10.5** for a summary). The actions may be **cognitive based**, e.g. something you would like to learn more about; they might be **based on feelings**, e.g. feel more confident in your use of a technique; or they may be focused on **the actual doing**, e.g. trying out different supervisory questions, setting up peer supervision sessions, or starting a conversation about organisational changes to supervision. We'd recommend an element of all three as you seek to identify your own personal development plan to enhance the effectiveness of your supervision practices and offer **Appendix 10.2** to record your thoughts.

We've asked you to think about what you would like to do, so in the spirit of working together, our final section will explore our aspirations for the 3Cs for Effective Supervision and some of the actions we have identified as our next priorities. We have identified these as essential to support the development of effective supervision for supervisees, for supervisors, but, of greatest importance, for the benefit of the people who access our services and all the people we will serve in the future.

TABLE 10.5 Overview of chapter contents to aid action planning

Chapter	Key content
1	Different types of supervision, purpose, and function, models and frameworks, sufficient time and safe spaces for supervision
2	Mindsets, motivation, appreciative, strengths-based approaches, learning and teaching principles
3	The importance of connections, content, and continuing development for effective supervision
4	Understanding yourself, your supervisee, the supervisory relationship, inclusivity
5	Practicalities of supervision, formats for supervision, processes, documentation
6	Preparing to be a supervisor or supervisee, reflection, active listening, feedback
7	Using occupational therapy knowledge and skills in supervision including groups, creative and coaching approaches
8	Performance evaluation, power and hierarchies, over- and underestimation of abilities of supervision
9	Quality assurance, managerial, organisational, and strategic perspectives of supervision
10	Future research and aspirations for supervision, action planning, implementing change

CRITICAL COMMENTARY

Our aspirations for supervision

In this final critical commentary, we are sharing our aspirations for supervision. Some ideas are within our influence and others we are capturing here but recognise it will take a whole-community approach to address them. So, thinking about each chapter, our aspirations for supervision look like this:

Chapter 1	International, national, and local policies are in place that recognise, value, and support supervision as an essential mechanism for safe and effective occupational therapy practices.
Chapter 2	That supervisors and supervisees adopt, and are supported to adopt, growth mindsets, appreciative, strengths-based approaches, and use learning and teaching principles to guide their supervision.
Chapter 3	The 3Cs for Effective Supervision are useful in enhancing supervisory practices for individuals, organisations, and the wider system.
Chapter 4	That people at all levels invest in and recognise the importance of the intra- and interpersonal relationships within supervision and their impact on safety, establishing trust, workforce retention, and wellbeing.
Chapter 5	That supervisors and supervisees are enabled to use formats, processes, and documentation to enhance their supervisory practice and journey.
Chapter 6	That supervision is universally recognised as a valued part of an occupational therapist's career from start to finish, and occupational therapists are supported to continuously update their knowledge and skills in effective supervisory practices.
Chapter 7	That occupational therapists leverage their professional knowledge and skills to enhance their supervisory practices.
Chapter 8	That supervisors and supervisees can enjoy and develop from the challenges that their supervision journey may offer them, and they are enabled and supported to do so.
Chapter 9	That effective supervision is seen as a strategic and organisational responsibility and critical for enhancing performance standards, valued as a safety mechanism, and acknowledged through formal structures and policies.
Chapter 10	We can build on the evidence base for supervision, implement changes to enhance supervision, and evaluate its impact for the profession, occupational therapists, organisations, and the people who access our services.

SUMMARY

We are excited by the potential of supervision that is yet to be fully realised in our profession. There is much work to be done to enhance supervision and we hope our offering of the 3Cs for Effective Supervision can be a useful part of this process. At times, we have written about individual 'Cs' within our framework, but it is important to remember they are interrelated and all of equal value. The 3Cs for Effective Supervision Framework will evolve as our thinking changes through critical engagement and reflection on supervision. We can already see that we need to represent the value of supervision not just within individual organisations but recognise the potential of high-quality professional development support when we look across settings, services, and countries. We see this book as the start of something, which hopefully will include more conversations with you.

If you are on social media, please use the **#3CSupervision** – we look forward to working together to further enhance effective supervision for occupational therapy.

REFERENCES

Aarons, G.A., Hurlburt, M., and Horwitz, S.M. (2011) 'Advancing a conceptual model of evidence-based practice implementation in public service sectors', *Administration and Policy in Mental Health and Mental Health Services*, 38(1), pp. 4–23. doi:10.1007/s10488-010-0327-7.

Atkins, L., Francis, J., Islam, R., O'Connor, D., Patey, A., Ivers, N., Foy, R., Duncan, E.M., Colquhoun, H., Grimshaw, H.M., Lawton, R., and Michie, S. (2017) 'A guide to using the Theoretical Domains Framework of behaviour change to investigate implementation problems', *Implementation Science*, 12(77), pp. 1–18. doi:10.1186/s13012-017-0605-9.

Balas, E.A. and Boren, S.A. (2000) 'Managing clinical knowledge for healthcare improvement', in van Bemmel, J. and McCray, A.T. (eds) *Yearbook of medical informatics*. New York, NY: Thieme, pp. 65–70.

Bartholomew Eldredge, L.K., Markham, C.M., Ruiter, R.A.C., Fernandez, M.E., Kok, G., and Parcel, G.S. (2016). *Planning health promotion programs: an intervention mapping approach*. San Francisco, CA: Jossey-Bass.

Brown, C.H., Curran, G., Palinkas, L.A., et al. (2017) 'An overview of research and evaluation designs for dissemination and implementation', *Annual Review of Public Health*, 38(1), 1–22. doi:10.1146/annurev-publhealth-031816-044215.

Chinman, M., Hunter, S.B., Ebener, P., Paddock, S.M., Stillman, L., Imm, P., and Wandersman, A. (2008) 'The Getting to Outcomes demonstration and evaluation: an illustration of the prevention support system', *American Journal of Community Psychology*, 41, pp. 206–224. doi:10.1007/s10464-008-9163-2.

Damschroder, L.J., Aron, D.C., Keith, R.E., Kirsh, S.R., Alexander, J.A., and Lowery, J.C. (2009) 'Fostering implementation of health services research findings into practice: a consolidated framework for advancing implementation science', *Implementation Science*, 4(1), pp. 1–15. doi:10.1186/1748-5908-4-50.

Dixon-Woods, M., McNicol, S., and Martin, G. (2012) 'Ten challenges in improving quality in healthcare: lessons from the Health Foundation's programme evaluations and relevant literature', *BMJ Quality & Safety*, 21, pp. 876–884. doi:10.1136/bmjqs-2011-000760.

Glasgow, R.E., Harden, S.M., Gaglio, B., Rabin, B., Smith, M.L., Porter, G.C., Ory, M.G., and Estabrooks, P.A. (2019) 'RE-AIM planning and evaluation framework: adapting to new science and practice with a 20-year review'. *Frontiers in Public Health*, 7, pp. 1–22. doi:10.3389/fpubh.2019.00064.

Glasgow, R.E., Vogt, T.M., and Boles, S.M. (1999) 'Evaluating the public health impact of health promotion interventions: the RE-AIM framework', *American Journal of Public Health*, 89, pp. 1322–1327. doi:10.2105/AJPH.89.9.1322.

Graham, F., Kennedy-Behr, A., and Ziviani, J. (2020) *Occupational performance coaching: a manual for practitioners and researchers*. Abingdon: Routledge.

Graham, I., Logan, J., Harrison, M., Straus, S., Tetroe, J., Caswell, W., and Robinson, N. (2006) 'Lost in knowledge translation: time for a map?' *Journal of Continuing Education in the Health Professions*, 26, pp. 13–24.

Handley, M.A., Gorukanti, A., and Cattamanchi, A. (2016) 'Strategies for implementing implementation science: a methodological overview', *Emergency Medicine Journal*, 33, pp. 660–664.

Hawkins, P. and McMahon, A. (2020) *Supervision in the helping professions*. 5th edn. London: Open University Press/McGraw Hill.

Ling, T., Bardsley, M., Adams, J., Lewis, R., and Roland, M. (2010) 'Evaluation of UK integrated care pilots: research protocol', *International Journal of Integrated Care*, 10(3), 1–15. doi:10.5334/ijic.513.

Martin, P., Lizarondo, L., Kumar, S., and Snowdon, D. (2021) 'Impact of clinical supervision on healthcare organisational outcomes: a mixed methods systematic review', *PLOS One*, 16(11), e0260156. doi:10.1371/journal.pone.0260156.

Metz, A. and Louison, L. (2018) *The Hexagon Tool: Exploring Context*. Chapel Hill, NC: National Implementation Research Network, Frank Porter Graham Child Development Institute, University of North Carolina at Chapel Hill. Available at: https://nirn.fpg.unc.edu (Accessed: 2 November 2021).

Meyers, D.C., Durlak, J.A., and Wandersman, A. (2012) 'The quality implementation framework: a synthesis of critical steps in the implementation process', *American Journal of Community Psychology*, 50(3–4), pp. 462–480. doi:10.1007/s10464-012-9522-x.

Moore, J.E. and Khan, S. (2020) *Designing for implementation course and workbook*. Available at: https://thecenterforimplementation.com/who-we-are.

Moullin, J.C., Dickson, K.S., Stadnick, N.A., Rabin, B., and Aarons, G.A. (2019) 'Systematic review of the Exploration, Preparation, Implementation, Sustainment (EPIS) Framework', *Implementation Science*, 14(1), pp. 1–16. doi:10.1186/s13012-018-0842-6.

Nilsen P. (2015) 'Making sense of implementation theories, models and frameworks', *Implementation Science*, 10(53), pp. 1–13. doi:10.1186/s13012-015-0242-0.

Powell, B.J., Waltz, T.J., Chinman, M.J., Damschroder, L.J., Smith, J.L., Matthieu, M.M., Proctor, E.K., and Kirchner, J.E. (2015) 'A refined compilation of implementation strategies: results from the Expert Recommendations for Implementing Change (ERIC) project', *Implementation Science*, 10(21), pp. 1–14. doi:10.1186/s13012-015-0209-1.

Proctor, E., Luke, D., Calhoun, A. et al. (2015) 'Sustainability of evidence-based healthcare: research agenda, methodological advances, and infrastructure support', *Implementation Science* 10(88), pp. 1–13. doi:10.1186/s13012-015-0274-5.

Proctor, E., Silmere, H., Raghavan, R., et al. (2011) 'Outcomes for implementation research: conceptual distinctions, measurement challenges, and research agenda', *Administration and Policy In Mental Health*, 38(2), pp. 65–76. doi:10.1007/s10488-010-0319-7.

Scheirer, M.A. (2005) 'Is sustainability possible? A review and commentary on empirical studies of program sustainability', *American Journal of Evaluation*, 26(3), pp. 320–347. doi:10.1177/1098214005278752.

Snowdon, D.A., Leggat, S.G., and Taylor, N.F. (2017) 'Does clinical supervision of healthcare professionals improve effectiveness of care and patient experience? A systematic review', *BMC Health Service Research*, 17, pp. 1–11. doi:10.1186/s12913-017-2739-5.

Stirman, S.W., Kimberly, J., Cook, N., Calloway, A., Castro, F., and Charns, M. (2012) 'The sustainability of new programs and innovations: a review of the empirical literature and recommendations for future research', *Implementation Science*, 7, pp. 1–19. doi:10.1186/1748-5908-7-17.

Wensing, M. and Grol, R. (2019) 'Knowledge translation in health: how implementation science could contribute more', *BMC Medicine*, 17(88), pp. 1–6. doi:10.1186/s12916-019-1322-9.

Appendix 10.1: Six Steps from Ideas to Implementation guidance template

1. WHAT IS HAPPENING NOW? WHAT WOULD IT LOOK LIKE IF IT WAS BETTER?	
• What needs to change? • How will you make the change? (Initial ideas only)	**Notes:**
2. WHAT CHANGE WOULD GET YOU CLOSER TO WHERE YOU WANT TO BE?	
• Clarify exactly what people will do differently by making an explicit list of required changes.	**Notes:**
3. WHO IS INVOLVED IN THIS CHANGE? WHO ARE YOUR ALLIES AND SUPPORTERS?	
• Who will be involved in creating and sustaining each change listed in point 2? Consider supervisors, supervisees, administrators, managers, others. • Who are your allies and supporters for this change?	**Notes:**

4. WHAT ARE THE BARRIERS AND FACILITATORS TO MAKING THIS CHANGE? WHAT IMPLEMENTATION STRATEGIES WILL TARGET THESE FACTORS?	
<ul><li>How will you find out what barriers and facilitators to change exist?</li><li>What behaviour change framework will you use to map the barriers and facilitators identified?</li><li>What are your key barriers and facilitators for change?</li><li>What are your implementation strategy options for addressing the barriers and leveraging the facilitators for change?</li></ul>	**Notes:**
5. WHAT OUTCOMES ARE EXPECTED? HOW WILL YOU KNOW CHANGE HAS HAPPENED?	
<ul><li>If the change was successful, what would you notice that was different?</li><li>What aspects of the change will you measure?</li><li>What evaluation tools/methods will you use?</li><li>When will you conduct the evaluation?</li></ul>	**Notes:**
6. HOW WILL YOU SUSTAIN AND/OR SCALE UP THE CHANGE?	
<ul><li>What options do you have for sustaining the change after the initial excitement has ended?</li><li>How might you embed the change into new workplace routines?</li><li>What adaptations to the intended change could happen/would be acceptable?</li><li>Is there an option for an implementation team to drive the change?</li></ul>	**Notes:**

Appendix 10.2: Actions to enhance supervision guidance template

For each chapter topic, note any actions that would enhance the effectiveness of yourself as a supervisee/supervisor, or the development of practices at operational or strategic levels. Actions may be **cognitive based**, e.g., learning something new; **based on feelings**, e.g., feel more confident in your use of a technique; or focused on **the actual doing**, e.g., setting up peer supervision, or initiating organisational changes to supervision.

Chapter 1 Different types of supervision, purpose, and function, models and frameworks, safe spaces
Chapter 2 Mindsets, motivation, appreciative, strengths-based approaches, learning and teaching principles

Chapter 3 The importance of connections, content, and continuing development for effective supervision

Chapter 4 Understanding yourself, your supervisee, the supervisory relationship, inclusivity

Chapter 5 Practicalities of supervision, formats for supervision, processes, documentation

Chapter 6 Preparing to be a supervisor or supervisee, reflection, active listening, feedback

Chapter 7 Using occupational therapy knowledge and skills in supervision including groups, creative and coaching approaches

Chapter 8 The potential impact of performance evaluation, power and hierarchies, over and underestimation of abilities on supervision

Chapter 9 Quality assurance, managerial, organisational, and strategic perspectives of supervision

Chapter 10 Future research and aspirations for supervision, action planning, implementing change

Index

Pages in *italics* refer to figures and **bold** refer to tables.

Printed in the United States
by Baker & Taylor Publisher Services

Printed in the United States
by Baker & Taylor Publisher Services